THE AUSTRALIAN
Women's Weekly

VEGETARIAN

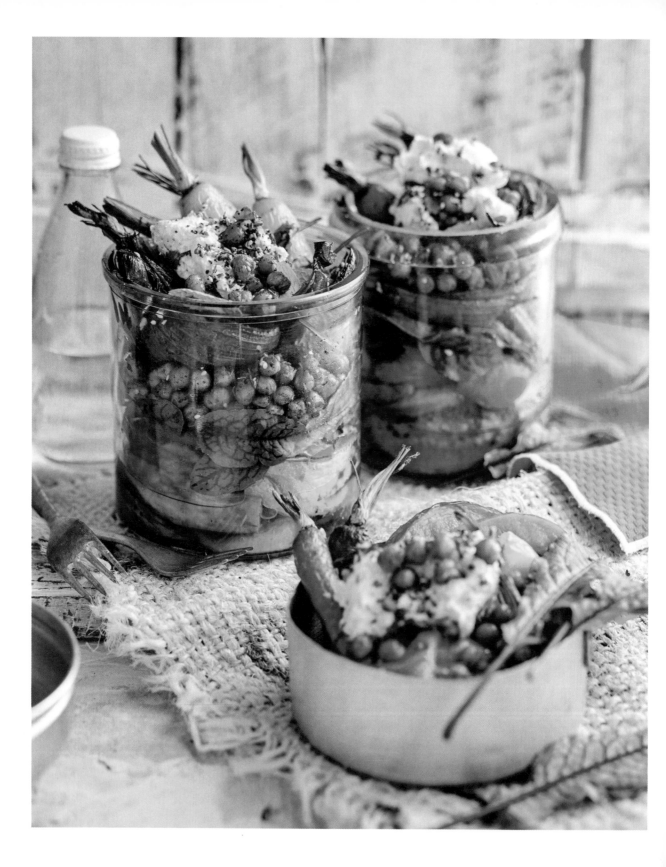

THE AUSTRALIAN Women's Weekly

VEGETARIAN

FLAVOURSOME, NUTRITIOUS EVERYDAY RECIPES

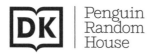

Project Editor Emma Hill
Project Designer Alison Shackleton
Editorial Assistant Kiron Gill
Jacket Designer Alison Donovan
Jackets Coordinator Lucy Philpott
Production Editor David Almond
Senior Producer Luca Bazzoli
Creative Technical Support Sonia Charbonnier
Managing Editor Dawn Henderson
Managing Art Editor Alison Donovan
Art Director Maxine Pedliham
Publishing Director Katie Cowan

Photographer Louise Lister
Stylist Emma Knowles
Photochefs Peta Dent, Amal Webster

First published in Great Britain in 2021
by Dorling Kindersley Limited
DK, One Embassy Gardens, 8 Viaduct Gardens, London, SW11 7BW

The authorised representative in the EEA is Dorling Kindersley
Verlag GmbH. Arnulfstr. 124, 80636 Munich, Germany

Copyright © 2021 Dorling Kindersley Limited
A Penguin Random House Company
10 9 8 7 6 5 4 3 2 1
001–324522–May/2021

A CIP catalogue record for this book is available from the British Library.
ISBN: 978-0-2415-1014-8

Printed and bound in China

For the curious
www.dk.com

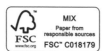

This book was made with Forest Stewardship Council ™ certified paper –
one small step in DK's commitment to a sustainable future.
For more information go to **www.dk.com/our-green-pledge**

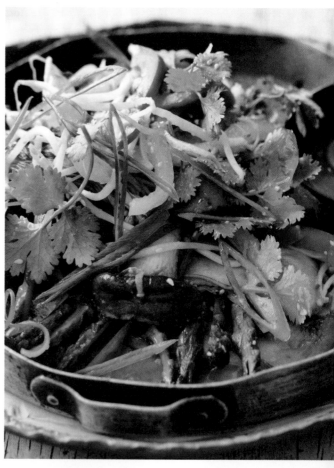

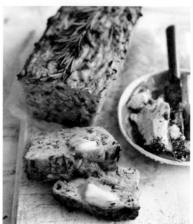

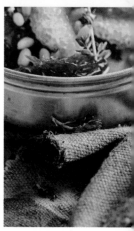

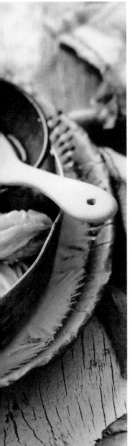
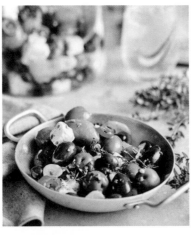
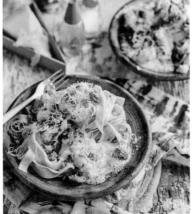

Contents

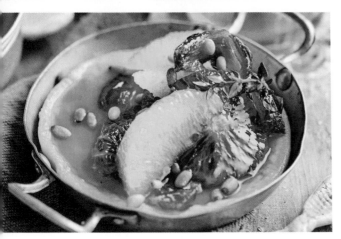

Plant-based pleasures

Vegetables. Fruit. Nuts. Seeds. Legumes. There is no shortage of delicious and fresh plant-based foods out there for us to enjoy. Whatever your reason for choosing meat-free meals, the advantages of vegetarianism and eating more plant foods are plenty and undeniable.

Why choose a vegetarian diet?

The percentage of people who enjoy a vegetarian diet has risen steadily over the years, but now more than ever, increasing numbers of people are taking interest in including more plant-based foods in their everyday diet. The importance of vegetarian foods, whether that be for health or environmental concerns, is now at the forefront of our minds.

A vegetarian diet is nothing new. There are many cultures and religions around the world that have practised vegetarianism for centuries, for traditional and ethical reasons. Modern vegetarians also have ethical reasons to avoid eating animals and animal products, including concern over the welfare of animals and the environmental impact of animal farming. Those who eat all or mostly plant foods leave the lightest footprint of us all on our fragile ecosystem and as we become more health conscious and socially aware about where our food comes from, going meat-free is becoming a mainstream choice.

Cutting out meat and animal products also has countless proven health benefits in a world where the over-consumption of processed meat is starting to take its toll on our bodies as well as the earth.

Studies have shown that those who eat a plant-based diet mostly live longer, carry less body fat, and are at a lower risk of developing type-2 diabetes, heart disease, digestive problems, and some cancers than those who consume a high proportion of meat. Even if you don't follow a strict vegetarian or vegan diet, there are still countless benefits to eating more meals that contain mostly or all plant-based foods.

The many faces of vegetarianism

Vegetarianism can be classed in a number of ways, so this book includes recipes for different types of vegetarian diet including lacto vegetarian for those who consume dairy but no meat, fish, or eggs; ovo vegetarian for people who eat eggs but no meat, fish, or dairy; lacto-ovo vegetarian for those who eat eggs and dairy but no meat or fish; and vegan for people who consume no meat, fish, egg, or dairy products.

Vegetarian food is now available in more places, options, flavours, and combinations than ever before – and in every cuisine. With an infinite variety of tastes and textures on offer, you can find endless ways to enjoy a varied, nutritious, and satisfying diet that is rich in vegetables and plant foods.

Maintaining a balanced diet

In many Western nations, vegetarians eat a diet that is closer to recommended nutritional intakes than omnivorous people. Vegetarian diets include higher percentages of dietary fibre from cereal foods, vegetables (including legumes), and fruits, providing the body with a better supply of the nutrition it requires to function optimally. With no meat intake, vegetarians also tend to consume less fat and salt overall, however, vegans and vegetarians should be mindful of eating foods that are high in saturated fat such as coconut oil and palm oil. It is possible to unbalance any diet by consuming too many dairy, fatty, or high sugar foods.

It can be easy for someone starting a vegetarian diet to over-compensate for the lack of meat with larger portions of processed carbohydrates. It is important instead to make sure you consume a wide variety of fruits, vegetables, seeds, nuts, and legumes so that you receive the full range of nutrients and minerals you need to keep healthy. A well-planned vegetarian diet should aim to easily fill all your daily nutritional requirements.

If you are following a vegan diet, it is even more essential that you take care to compensate for the absence of the nutrients you would usually get from animal products. It is especially important for anyone on a plant-based diet to follow recommended portion sizes for all food groups in order to maintain the best balance for your body.

Meeting nutritional needs

While most sources of nutrients can be found by eating a varied plant-based diet, there are some key nutritional needs that vegans and vegetarians should take particular care to meet in order to avoid any issues that can be caused by deficiencies. Here are some of the most commonly missed nutrients for vegetarians and where they can be found:

CALCIUM Dairy products, nuts, seeds, beans, soy products, dark leafy green vegetables, fortified unsweetened rice and oat drinks.

IODINE Small amounts of iodised salt, sea vegetables such as nori, wakame, or kombu.

IRON Nuts, soy products, lentils, oats, dried fruits, dark leafy green vegetables – eat with vitamin C-rich foods to help the body absorb the iron.

OMEGA-3 FATTY ACIDS Eggs, flaxseeds, chia seeds, pepitas (pumpkin seeds), walnuts, seaweed.

PROTEIN Whole grains, legumes, eggs, dairy products, nuts, seeds, soy products.

VITAMIN B12 There is no plant food that contains sufficient levels of B12, so vegetarians and vegans in particular should look to include foods fortified with B12 or take a supplement as part of a balanced diet.

VITAMIN C Tomatoes, red capsicum (peppers), citrus fruit, broccoli, berries.

VITAMIN D Fortified foods, vitamin D supplements, exposure to sunlight (take care to protect the skin).

ZINC Whole grains, nuts, pepitas (pumpkin seeds), wheatgerm, soy products.

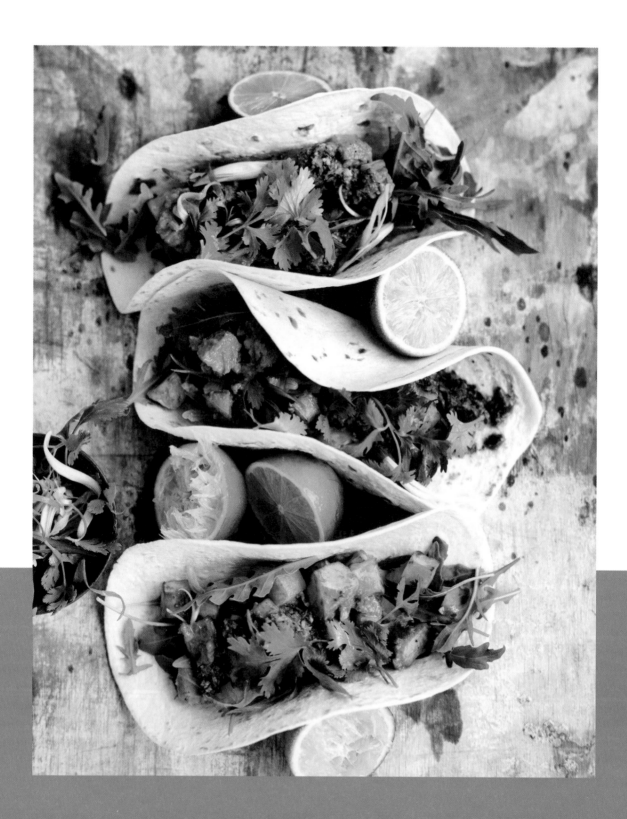

ON THE LIGHT SIDE

Perfect for lunchtime or a light supper, these inventive veggie dishes are packed with nutritious health-giving ingredients and bold flavours.

Roasted vegetables with basil and feta polenta

LACTO VEGETARIAN | PREP + COOK TIME **50 MINUTES** | SERVES **6**

An Italian storecupboard staple, polenta is made of ground cornmeal and can be fried, baked, or served as a creamy mash. It makes a great substitute for rice or pasta and works well as a hearty base for vegetarian dishes.

500g butternut pumpkin (butternut squash), coarsely chopped

2 large courgettes (300g), coarsely chopped

2 medium red onions (340g), quartered

2 large red capsicums (peppers) (700g), coarsely chopped

1 tbsp cumin seeds

2 tsp ground coriander

$^1/_2$ tsp dried chilli flakes

2 garlic cloves, crushed

$^1/_4$ cup (60ml) olive oil

salt and freshly ground black pepper

2 tbsp red wine vinegar

1.5 litres (6 cups) vegetable stock

$1^1/_2$ cups (250g) polenta

200g Danish feta, crumbled

$^1/_2$ cup (10g) torn fresh basil leaves

$^1/_3$ cup (45g) coarsely chopped toasted hazelnuts

1 Preheat oven to 220°C (200°C fan/425°F/Gas 7). Line two large oven trays with baking paper.

2 Combine the pumpkin, courgette, onion, capsicum, cumin, coriander, chilli, garlic, and olive oil in a large bowl; season with salt and pepper. Place the vegetables on the trays; roast for 30 minutes or until golden and tender. Drizzle with vinegar.

3 Meanwhile, bring the stock to the boil in a large saucepan. Gradually add the polenta, whisking continuously. Reduce heat; simmer, stirring, for 10 minutes or until the polenta thickens. Stir in 125g of the feta and $^1/_3$ cup (7g) of the basil.

4 Serve the polenta immediately, topped with the vegetables, hazelnuts, remaining feta, and remaining basil.

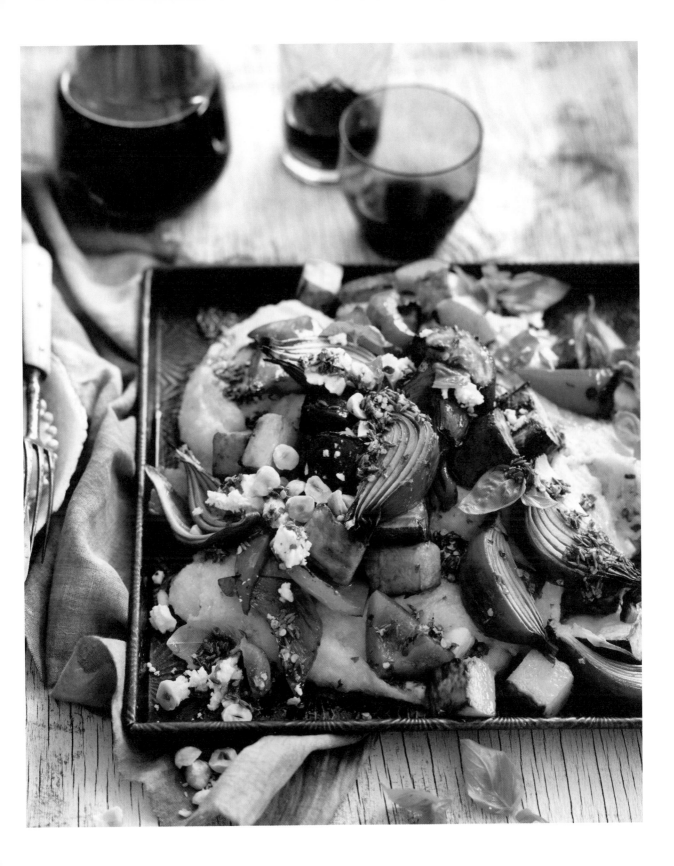

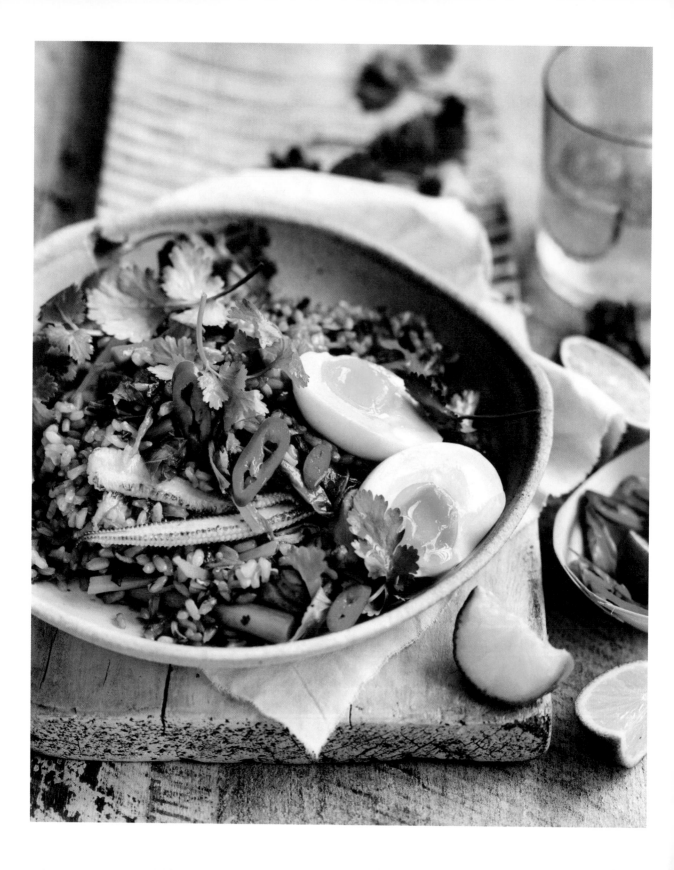

Brown rice nasi goreng

OVO VEGETARIAN | PREP + COOK TIME **45 MINUTES** | SERVES **4**

Nasi goreng is a traditional dish from Indonesia and translates as "fried rice". Indonesian cooks typically use whatever ingredients they have to hand combined with leftover rice from the previous day. Serve with sambal – a chilli sauce – for an authentic kick.

400g gai lan (Chinese broccoli)

375g choy sum

$^1/_2$ cup (8g) fresh coriander leaves

4 eggs

2 tbsp peanut oil

6 shallots (150g), halved, thinly sliced

4cm piece fresh ginger, cut into thin matchsticks

2 garlic cloves, crushed

2 fresh long red chillies, thinly sliced

150g button mushrooms, quartered

100g shiitake mushrooms, thinly sliced

115g baby corn, halved lengthways

$3^1/_2$ cups (625g) cooked brown rice (see tip)

2 tbsp kecap manis

1 tsp sesame oil

salt and freshly ground black pepper

lime wedges, to serve

1 Cut the stalks from the gai lan and choy sum. Cut stalks into 10cm lengths; cut leaves into 10cm pieces. Keep the stalks and leaves separated. Chop half the coriander; reserve the remaining leaves.

2 Cook the eggs in a medium saucepan of boiling water for 5 minutes or until soft-boiled; drain. When cool enough to handle, peel the eggs.

3 Meanwhile, heat half the peanut oil in a wok over a medium heat; stir-fry the shallots for 8 minutes or until soft and light golden. Add the ginger, garlic, and half the chilli; stir-fry for 4 minutes or until softened. Transfer the mixture to a plate.

4 Heat the remaining peanut oil in a wok over a medium-high heat; stir-fry the mushrooms and baby corn for 4 minutes or until just tender. Add the gai lan and choy sum stalks; stir-fry for 3 minutes. Add the gai lan and choy sum leaves, cooked rice, kecap manis, sesame oil, shallot mixture, and chopped coriander; stir-fry for 3 minutes or until the rice is hot and the leaves are wilted. Season with salt and pepper to taste.

5 Top the nasi goreng with the eggs, reserved coriander leaves, and the remaining chilli. Serve with lime wedges.

TIP

You will need to cook 1½ cups (300g) brown rice for the amount of cooked rice needed in this recipe.

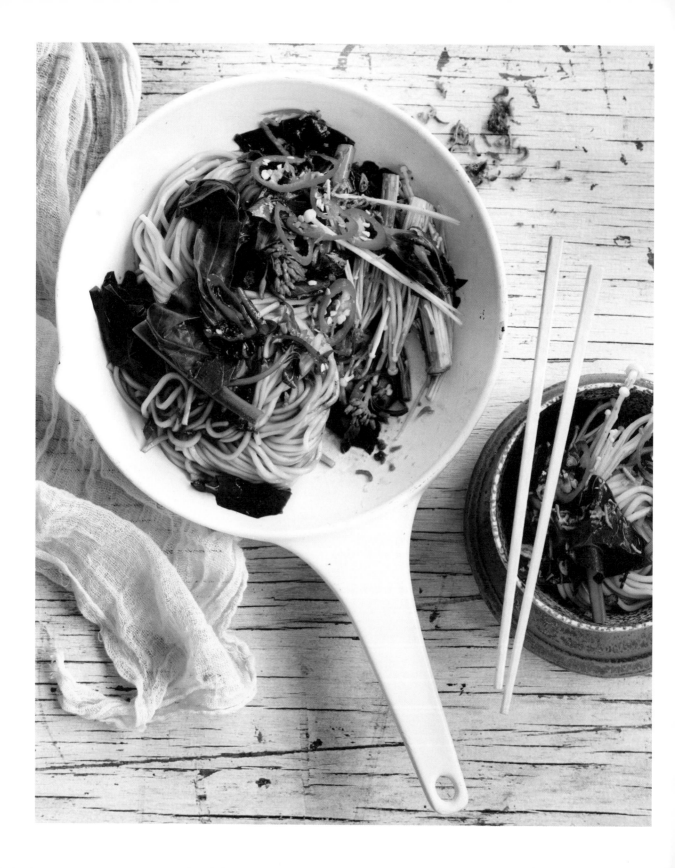

Gai lan and mushroom five-spice stir-fry

VEGAN | PREP + COOK TIME **20 MINUTES** | SERVES **4**

Chinese five-spice is a mixture of cinnamon, cloves, fennel seeds, star anise, and Sichuan pepper. It encompasses all of the key flavours of Asian cooking – sweet, sour, bitter, salty, and umami – and brings fragrance and complexity to a range of dishes.

450g thin udon noodles

430g gai lan (Chinese broccoli)

2 tbsp peanut oil

2 garlic cloves, crushed

1 fresh long red chilli, thinly sliced

1/2 tsp Chinese five-spice

2 tbsp vegetarian oyster sauce (see tips)

2 tbsp kecap manis

1/2 tsp sesame oil

200g enoki mushrooms, trimmed

2 tbsp fried Asian shallots (see tips)

1 Place the noodles in a medium heatproof bowl with enough boiling water to cover, separate with a fork; drain.

2 Separate the gai lan stalks and leaves; chop coarsely, keeping the stalks and leaves separate.

3 Heat the peanut oil in a wok over a high heat; stir-fry the garlic and half the chilli for 2 minutes or until softened. Add the five-spice and gai lan stalks; stir-fry for 1 minute or until tender.

4 Add the oyster sauce, kecap manis, sesame oil, and noodles; stir-fry for 1 minute or until hot. Add the gai lan leaves; cook for a further 1 minute. Toss through the mushrooms.

5 Serve the stir-fry topped with the shallots and remaining chilli.

TIPS

- While regular oyster sauce is made from oysters and their brine, the vegetarian version is instead made from mushrooms.
- Fried shallots are available from Asian food stores and some supermarkets. Or you can make your own by frying thinly sliced peeled shallots until golden-brown and crisp.

Japanese cabbage pancakes

OVO VEGETARIAN | PREP + COOK TIME **50 MINUTES + STANDING** | SERVES **4**

These quick cabbage pancakes are known as okonomiyaki in Japan, where they are enjoyed as street food. They consist of batter and cabbage but the toppings traditionally vary greatly so feel free to add any leftover vegetables you like.

1³/₄ cups (255g) plain flour

¹/₃ cup (50g) cornflour

2 eggs

1¹/₂ cups (375ml) water

6 cups (480g) finely shredded cabbage

¹/₃ cup (90g) pink pickled ginger

2 tbsp sesame oil

2 green onions (spring onions), thinly sliced

pink pickled ginger, extra, to serve

1 tbsp sesame seeds, toasted

dipping sauce

¹/₄ cup (60ml) light soy sauce

1 tbsp rice wine vinegar

2 tsp sesame oil

1 Whisk the flour, cornflour, eggs, and water in a large bowl until smooth and combined; stand for 15 minutes.

2 Meanwhile, preheat oven to 130°C (110°C fan/250°F/Gas¹/₂). Line an oven tray with baking paper.

3 To make the dipping sauce, combine the ingredients in a small bowl.

4 Add the cabbage and ginger to the batter; stir to combine.

5 Heat 2 teaspoons of the sesame oil in a large frying pan over a medium heat. Spoon one quarter of the batter mixture into the pan, flattening to form a 2.5cm thick pancake; cook the pancake for 4 minutes each side or until golden and cooked through. Transfer to the oven tray; keep warm in oven. Repeat the process with the remaining oil and batter to make four pancakes in total.

6 Top the pancakes with green onion, the extra pickled ginger, and sesame seeds; serve with the dipping sauce.

TIP

Traditional condiments served with okonomiyaki are Japanese mayonnaise and spicy barbecue sauce (as pictured).

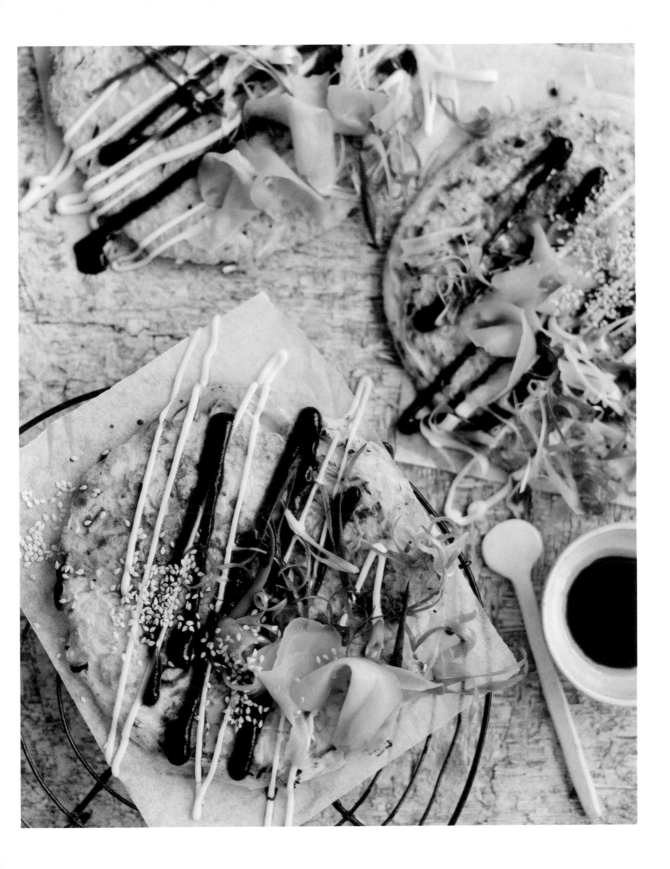

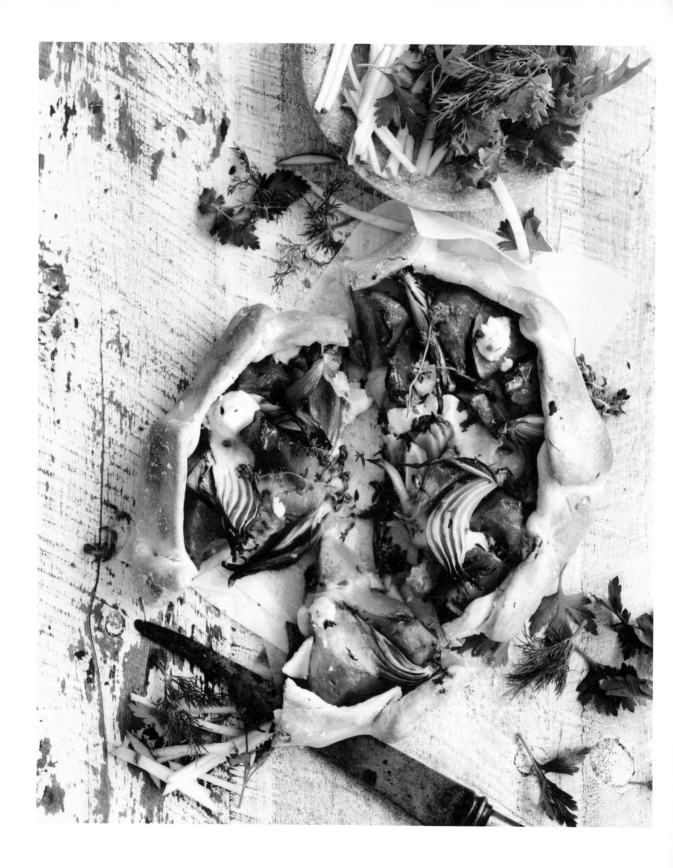

Pumpkin and feta free-form tart

LACTO-OVO VEGETARIAN | PREP + COOK TIME **1 HOUR 30 MINUTES + REFRIGERATION** | SERVES **4**

To make a free-form tart the pastry dough is laid flat on an oven tray rather than being placed in a tart tin. The filling is then arranged in the centre and the pastry edges are folded around it, resulting in a pleasingly rustic finish. Swap pumpkin for sweet potato, if you like.

800g Japanese pumpkin (kabocha squash),
cut into 3cm pieces

2 medium red onions (340g), cut into wedges

2 tsp fresh thyme leaves

1 tbsp olive oil

salt and freshly ground black pepper

80g feta, crumbled

2 bocconcini (70g), torn

2 tbsp fresh thyme

cream cheese pastry

1¼ cups (185g) plain flour

½ tsp sea salt flakes

125g cold cream cheese, chopped

1 free-range egg

1 tbsp cold water, approximately

mixed leaf salad

100g baby mixed salad leaves

½ cup (10g) coarsely chopped fresh flat-leaf parsley

1 tbsp fresh dill sprigs

1 medium beurre bosc pear (230g), cut into matchsticks

1 tbsp olive oil

1 tbsp lemon juice

1   Preheat oven to 200°C (180°C fan/400°F/Gas 6).

2   Place the pumpkin, onion, and thyme on a baking-paper-lined oven tray; drizzle with olive oil. Season with salt and pepper. Bake for 25 minutes or until tender. Cool.

3   Meanwhile, make the cream cheese pastry. Process the flour, salt, and cream cheese until crumbly; add the egg and the water, pulse until mixture just comes together. Knead the dough on a floured surface until smooth. Wrap in plastic wrap (cling film); refrigerate for 20 minutes.

4   Roll the pastry between sheets of baking paper to a 30cm round. Remove the top sheet of baking paper; lift pastry on the paper to a second oven tray. Top the pastry with the pumpkin mixture, feta, and bocconcini, leaving a 4cm border all around. Fold the pastry sides over the filling, pleating as you go to partially cover.

5   Bake the tart for 30 minutes or until golden and the base is cooked through.

6   Meanwhile, make the mixed leaf salad. Place the ingredients in a large bowl; toss gently to combine. Season with salt and pepper to taste.

7   Top the tart with the thyme and serve with salad.

Roasted sticky tofu buns

VEGAN | PREP + COOK TIME **45 MINUTES + STANDING** | SERVES **4**

Tofu is rich in protein, low in fat, and 100 per cent plant-based. It is often seasoned or marinated to enhance the dish it stars in, and due to its porous texture it absorbs flavours beautifully. This recipe can easily be doubled or tripled to feed more people.

300g firm tofu

1 tsp smoked paprika

salt and freshly ground black pepper

1½ tbsp tomato sauce (ketchup)

1½ tbsp smoky barbecue sauce

¼ cup (60ml) soy sauce

¼ cup (60ml) rice wine vinegar

2 tbsp brown sugar

1 cucumber (130g), thinly sliced lengthways

1 large carrot (180g), thinly sliced lengthways

1 fresh long red chilli, thinly sliced on the diagonal

1 tbsp caster sugar

2 tbsp rice wine vinegar, extra

4 fresh coriander sprigs

1 tbsp coarsely chopped roasted salted peanuts

4 small soft white bread rolls, split

1 Preheat oven to 200°C (180°C fan/400°F/Gas 6). Grease and line an oven tray with baking paper.

2 Place the tofu on a plate lined with paper towel. Top with another plate; stand for 10 minutes. Cut the tofu crossways into eight slices, rub with paprika; season with salt and pepper.

3 Bring the tomato sauce, barbecue sauce, soy sauce, vinegar, and brown sugar to a simmer in a small saucepan over a medium heat. Simmer for 3 minutes or until thickened slightly. Pour the sauce mixture over the tofu; turn to coat. Transfer the tofu to the tray; bake for 20 minutes or until the tofu is golden, basting occasionally with the sauce mixture.

4 Combine the cucumber, carrot, chilli, caster sugar, and extra vinegar in a medium bowl; stand for 10 minutes or until the vegetables soften. Drain.

5 Place the tofu, pickled vegetables, coriander, and nuts in the split rolls.

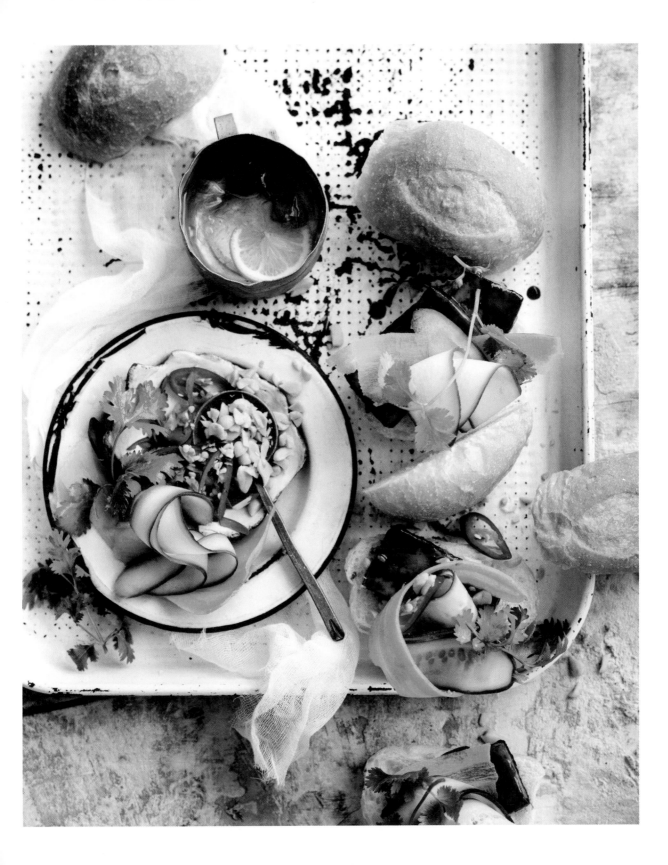

Cauliflower burger

LACTO-OVO VEGETARIAN | PREP + COOK TIME **40 MINUTES + REFRIGERATION** | MAKES **4**

The combination of cauliflower, beetroot, and cannellini beans in this veggie classic makes for a brilliant burger texture that holds its shape perfectly, plus it's super nutritious. To make it even tastier serve with a generous drizzle of homemade lemon mayonnaise.

350g beetroot, peeled, coarsely grated

1 small red onion (100g), thinly sliced

1 tsp salt flakes

1/4 cup (60ml) red wine vinegar

1 tbsp brown sugar

2 tbsp chopped fresh thyme

250g cauliflower, coarsely chopped

140g piece vegetarian cheddar

1/2 cup (100g) canned cannellini beans, drained, rinsed

1 cup (70g) fresh breadcrumbs

2 tbsp chopped fresh flat-leaf parsley

2 tsp finely grated lemon rind

2 tbsp skinless chopped hazelnuts, toasted

salt and freshly ground black pepper

1 free-range egg white, lightly beaten

2 tbsp vegetable oil

8 large butter (round) lettuce leaves

125g cherry heirloom tomatoes, halved

lemon mayonnaise

1/3 cup (100g) whole-egg mayonnaise

2 tsp finely grated lemon rind

2 tsp lemon juice

salt and freshly ground black pepper

1 Place the beetroot, onion, salt, vinegar, sugar, and thyme in a medium saucepan; bring to the boil. Reduce heat; simmer, stirring occasionally, for 20 minutes or until the beetroot is tender and slightly sticky. Cool.

2 Meanwhile, boil, steam, or microwave the cauliflower until tender. Drain; cool. Slice 90g of the vegetarian cheddar into 4 thin slices; grate the remaining cheddar.

3 Place the cauliflower and beans in a food processor, pulse until coarsely chopped (do not over process). Transfer to a large bowl. Add 1/4 cup (15g) of the breadcrumbs, the grated vegetarian cheddar, parsley, lemon rind, and hazelnuts; season with salt and pepper, stir to combine. Shape the cauliflower mixture into four patties. Refrigerate for 30 minutes.

4 Make the lemon mayonnaise. Whisk the ingredients in a small bowl until combined; season with salt and pepper to taste.

5 Dip the patties in the egg white; coat patties in remaining breadcrumbs.

6 Heat the vegetable oil in a large frying pan over a medium-high heat; cook the patties for 4 minutes each side or until browned and crisp. Drain on paper towel. Immediately top with the sliced cheese for the cheese to melt.

7 Place each patty in a lettuce leaf; top with the tomato and a generous spoonful of the beetroot mixture (you will only use half the mixture, see tip). Drizzle with lemon mayonnaise; top with the remaining lettuce leaf.

TIP

Refrigerate leftover beetroot mixture in an airtight container for up to 1 week.

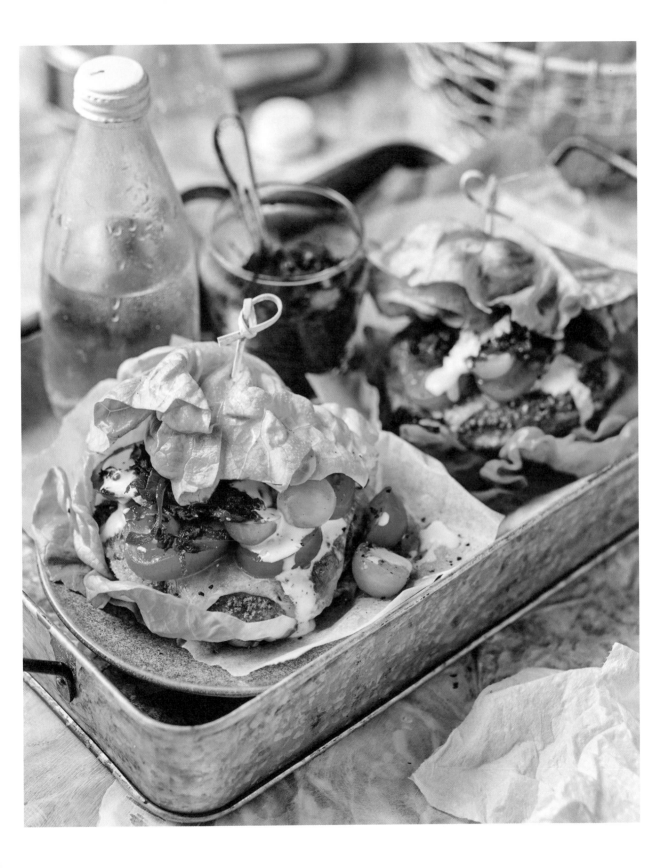

Grilled vegetable and capsicum relish subs

OVO VEGETARIAN | PREP + COOK TIME **50 MINUTES + COOLING** | SERVES **4**

This capsicum relish is good enough to stand alone as a zingy dip for crackers or crudités and will perk up any grilled sandwich. For a gluten-free variation on this recipe serve the vegetables, relish, and aïoli in lettuce cups.

2 baby aubergines (130g), cut into 1cm slices

200g patty pan squash, cut into 1cm slices

200g butternut pumpkin (butternut squash), thinly sliced

cooking-oil spray

salt and freshly ground black pepper

4 mini baguette rolls (680g)

$1/3$ cup (100g) aïoli

$1/2$ cup (8g) fresh coriander sprigs

capsicum relish

1 tbsp olive oil

1 small brown onion (80g), finely chopped

1 garlic clove, crushed

1 tsp ground cumin

$1/2$ tsp chilli powder

2 medium red capsicums (peppers) (400g), coarsely chopped

2 medium yellow capsicums (peppers) (400g), coarsely chopped

2 tbsp brown sugar

2 tbsp red wine vinegar

1 To make the capsicum relish, heat the olive oil in a medium frying pan over a medium heat; cook the onion, garlic, and spices, covered, for 5 minutes. Add the capsicum; cook, covered, for 20 minutes, stirring occasionally, or until soft. Stir in the sugar and vinegar; cook until syrupy. Cool.

2 Meanwhile, spray the aubergine, squash, and pumpkin with the cooking-oil spray; season with salt and pepper. Cook the vegetables in batches, on a heated oiled grill plate (or grill or barbecue) over a medium-high heat for 3 minutes each side or until browned and tender.

3 Split the rolls in half. Spread each roll with 1 tablespoon of aïoli; top with the vegetables, relish, and coriander.

TIP

Capsicum relish can be kept refrigerated in an airtight container for up to 1 week.

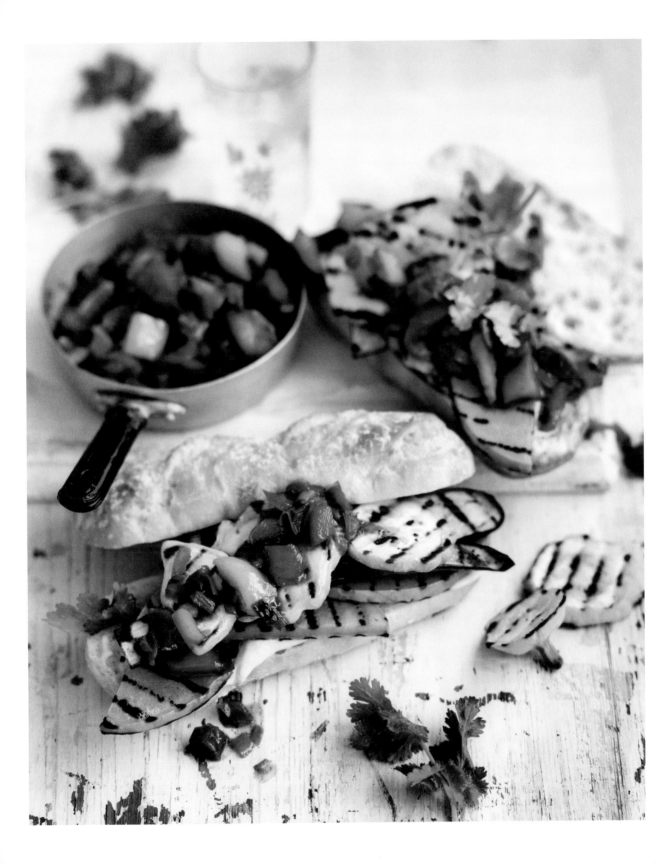

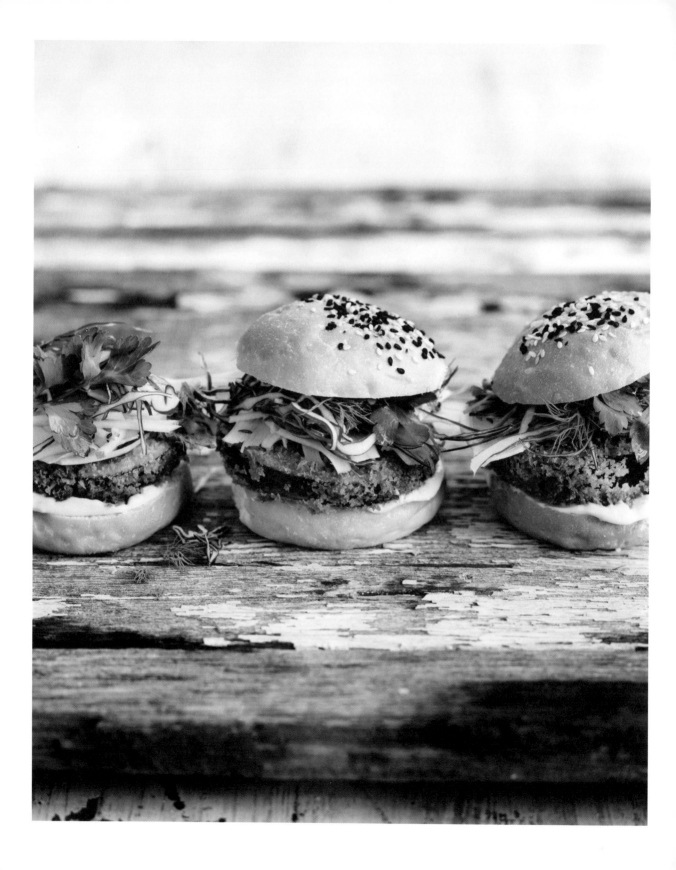

Aubergine schnitzel buns

LACTO-OVO VEGETARIAN | PREP + COOK TIME **45 MINUTES** | MAKES **6**

With a meltingly soft interior and a crunchy breadcrumb crust, these aubergine schnitzels
are an instant crowd-pleaser. For speed and simplicity you could use panko (Japanese)
breadcrumbs instead of making your own.

300g stale sourdough bread, coarsely torn

1 large aubergine (500g)

1/2 cup (75g) plain flour

2 eggs, lightly beaten

2 tbsp olive oil

60g butter, coarsely chopped

6 brioche buns (540g)

1/4 cup (75g) aïoli

apple slaw

1/4 cup (60ml) buttermilk

1 tbsp olive oil

2 tsp dijon mustard

1 tbsp lemon juice

salt and freshly ground black pepper

1 tsp caraway seeds, toasted, coarsely crushed

2 cups (160g) shredded purple cabbage

1/2 medium red apple (75g), cut into matchsticks

1/2 baby fennel bulb (65g), thinly sliced, fronds
reserved

1 cup (60g) fresh flat-leaf parsley leaves

1   To make the apple slaw, combine the buttermilk, olive oil, mustard, and
    lemon juice in a large bowl; season with salt and pepper to taste. Add the
    caraway seeds, cabbage, apple, fennel, reserved fronds, and parsley; toss
    to gently combine.

2   Process the sourdough until fine crumbs form; transfer to an oven tray.
    Trim the top from the aubergine; cut the aubergine into 6 thick rounds.
    Coat the aubergine in flour; shake away excess. Dip the aubergine in the
    egg mixture, then coat in the breadcrumbs.

3   Preheat oven to 130°C (110°C fan/250°F/Gas 1/2). Line an oven tray with
    baking paper.

4   Heat half the oil and half the butter in a large frying pan over medium-
    high; cook the aubergine for 2 minutes each side or until golden and
    cooked through. Transfer to an oven tray; keep warm in oven. Repeat
    frying with the remaining oil, butter, and aubergine.

5   Split the buns in half. Spread bun bases with aïoli; top with aubergine
    apple slaw, and bun tops.

TIP

We used Pink Lady apples in this recipe, or you
could use a green variety.

Green quinoa with sesame eggs

OVO VEGETARIAN | PREP + COOK TIME **25 MINUTES** | SERVES **2**

Quinoa is a nutritious wheat-free alternative to starchy grains with numerous health benefits
that have caused its popularity to soar in recent years. It's packed with fibre, protein,
vitamins, and minerals making it the perfect addition to a vegetarian diet.

1 cup (250g) vegetable stock

1/2 cup (100g) white quinoa, rinsed

4 eggs, at room temperature

2 tsp coconut oil

1 small garlic clove, crushed

1 fresh small red chilli, thinly sliced

2 cups (80g) thinly sliced kale (see tip)

2 cups (90g) firmly packed, thinly sliced silverbeet
(swiss chard) (see tip)

1 tbsp lemon juice

salt and freshly ground black pepper

1/4 cup (5g) finely chopped fresh flat-leaf parsley

1 tbsp white sesame seeds

1 tbsp black sesame seeds

1 tsp sea salt flakes

1 Place the stock and quinoa in a medium saucepan; bring to the boil.
Reduce heat to low-medium; simmer gently, for 15 minutes or until most
of the stock is absorbed. Remove from heat; cover, stand for 5 minutes.

2 Meanwhile, cook the eggs in a small saucepan of boiling water for
5 minutes. Remove immediately from the boiling water; cool under
running cold water for 30 seconds.

3 Heat the coconut oil in a medium saucepan over a medium heat. Add
the garlic and chilli; cook, stirring, for 2 minutes or until fragrant.
Add the kale and silverbeet; stir until wilted. Add the cooked quinoa
and lemon juice; season with salt and pepper to taste.

4 Combine the parsley, both sesame seeds, and salt in a small bowl.
Peel the eggs; roll in the parsley mixture.

5 Serve quinoa topped with eggs.

TIP

Leftover greens can be wilted in a little olive oil
or chopped and added to soups.

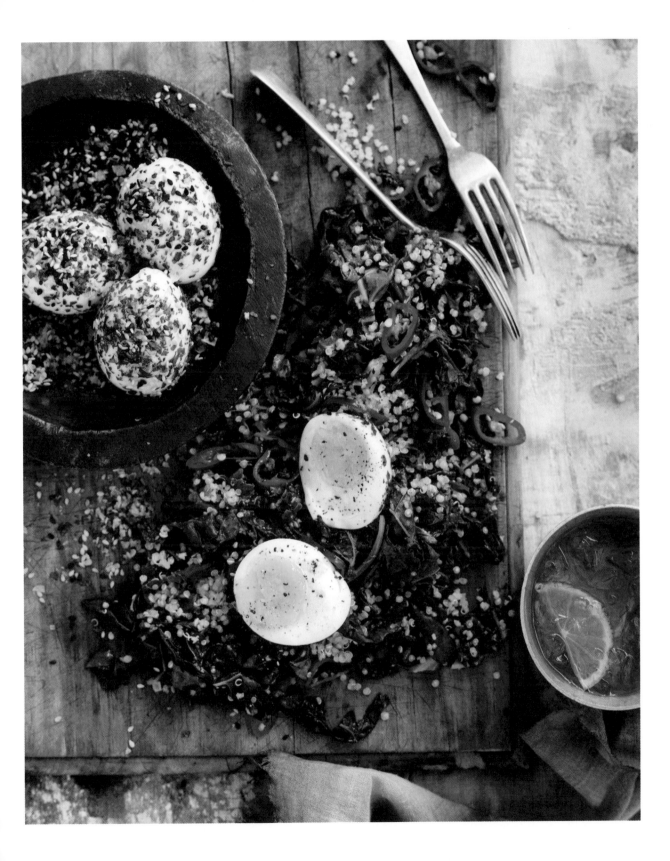

Vegetable larb

VEGAN | PREP + COOK TIME **45 MINUTES** | SERVES **4**

Traditional larb is a tangy salad of minced pork (or chicken) and fresh herbs, originating from Laos but also found in northern Thailand. This vegan version keeps the traditional flavours and instead mixes them with the crisp textures of raw vegetables.

1/4 cup (60ml) tamari

1/4 cup (60ml) lime juice

1/2 tsp dried chilli flakes

1 large beetroot (200g), peeled, cut into 5mm pieces

2 medium carrots (240g), unpeeled, cut into 5mm pieces

250g snake beans, cut into 5mm pieces (see tip)

2 cucumbers (230g), halved lengthways

1/3 cup (65g) jasmine rice

250g baby roma (plum) tomatoes, halved

5 green onions (spring onions), thinly sliced

2/3 cup (4g) finely chopped fresh mint

1/4 cup (5g) finely chopped fresh Thai basil or coriander

1/2 cup (70g) roasted unsalted peanuts, finely chopped

1 medium butter (round) lettuce, leaves separated

lime wedges, to serve

1 Preheat oven to 180°C (160°C fan/350°F/Gas 4).

2 Combine tamari, lime juice, and chilli flakes in a large bowl.

3 Combine beetroot and 1½ tablespoons of the dressing in a small bowl. Combine the carrot, snake beans, and ¼ cup (60ml) of the dressing in a medium bowl. Remove seeds from the cucumber; cut into 5mm pieces. Add the cucumber to the remaining dressing in large bowl. Cover each bowl with plastic wrap (cling film); stand vegetables for 15 minutes.

4 Meanwhile, place the rice on an oven tray; roast for 12 minutes or until golden. Process the rice in a small food processor (or crush with a mortar and pestle) until very finely chopped.

5 Add the tomatoes to the cucumber mixture with the green onion, herbs, ground rice, carrot mixture, and half the peanuts. Strain the beetroot mixture through a sieve, add to the larb; toss gently to combine.

6 Serve the larb with lettuce leaves and lime wedges, sprinkled with the remaining peanuts.

TIP

Snake beans can be found in some Asian food stores. Alternatively, French beans can be used as a substitute.

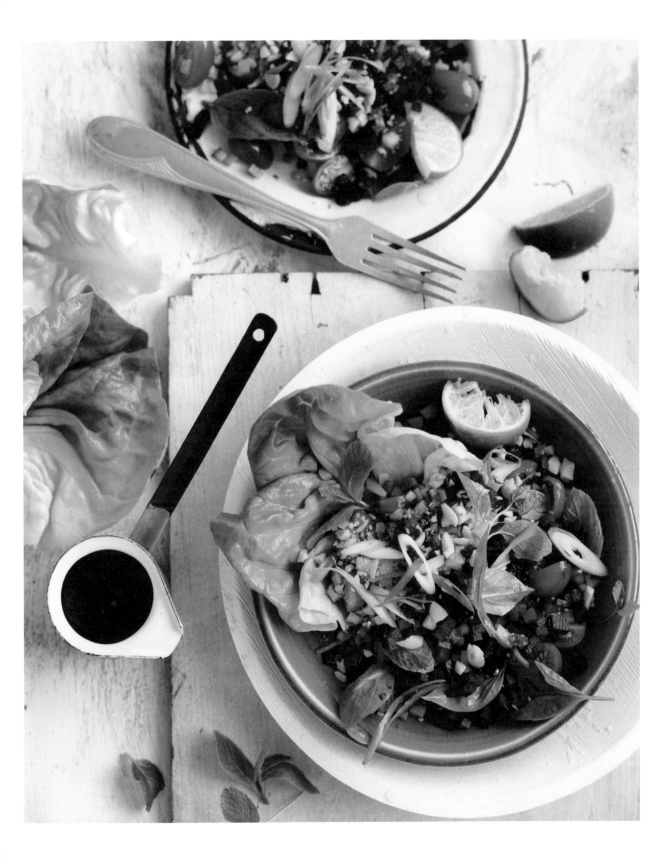

Tofu

VEGAN

Tofu is a great source of plant-based protein that can be used in all sorts of ways, so is a fantastic ingredient to bring nutritious variety to a vegetarian or vegan diet. You can stir-fry it, add it to your favourite curries, soups, salads, and even smoothies.

Breakfast super scramble

VEGAN | PREP + COOK TIME **10 MINUTES** | SERVES **2**

Coarsely break up 250g firm tofu with a fork. Heat 2 tablespoons of olive oil in a large frying pan; cook 2 chopped green onions (spring onions), stirring, for 1 minute or until softened. Add the tofu and 2 tablespoons of sriracha sauce; cook, stirring, over a high heat for 2 minutes. Add 1 cup (40g) of coarsely chopped baby kale leaves; season with salt and pepper, stir until wilted and heated through. Serve sprinkled with 2 tablespoons of toasted sesame seeds. To make this even heartier, stir in a drained and crushed 400g can of kidney beans and a handful of coriander sprigs.

Baked tofu yumminess

VEGAN | PREP + COOK TIME **45 MINUTES** | SERVES **2**

Preheat oven to 220°C (200°C fan/425°F/Gas 7). Cut 300g of firm tofu into 1cm thick slices, place between sheets of paper towel; weigh down with a chopping board, for 5 minutes. Combine $^1/_3$ cup (80ml) hoisin sauce, ½ teaspoon of Chinese five spice, and 1 teaspoon each of sesame oil and rice wine vinegar in a small bowl. Place tofu slices, one at a time, into the sauce mixture, turning to coat; place on a baking-paper-lined oven tray. Bake for 30 minutes or until golden and caramelized. Serve warm tofu in buns layered with thinly sliced carrot, cucumber, green onion (spring onions), red chilli, and coriander.

Raspberry thickshake

VEGAN | PREP TIME **10 MINUTES** | SERVES **2** MAKES **2 CUPS (500ML)**

Blend 300g firm silken tofu with a 2cm piece of fresh ginger, 150g of frozen raspberries, and $^1/_4$ cup (60ml) of pure maple syrup until smooth. Add a tray of ice-cubes; blend until smooth. Serve topped with chopped roasted cashews and extra frozen raspberries.

Tofu miso baked pumpkin soup

VEGAN | PREP + COOK TIME **1 HOUR 30 MINUTES** MAKES **7 CUPS (1.75 LITRES)**

Preheat oven to 220°C (200°C fan/425°F/Gas 7). Place 2 unpeeled medium (300g) brown onions and half an unpeeled, unseeded butternut pumpkin (butternut squash) (1.3kg) on a baking-paper-lined oven tray; score the pumpkin flesh in a criss-cross pattern, top with 1 tablespoon each of olive oil and honey. Cover with foil; roast for 45 minutes. Remove foil; roast for 30 minutes or until pumpkin is tender. Discard pumpkin seeds and the skins from the onions. Scoop pumpkin flesh into a blender, add the onion, $^1/_3$ cup (80ml) white (shiro) miso, 2 tablespoons of lemon juice and 300g of firm silken tofu; blend until smooth. Pour the mixture into a saucepan with 3 cups (750ml) of vegetable stock; season. Stir until heated through. Top with coriander. Serve with grilled pitta bread.

CLOCKWISE from top left

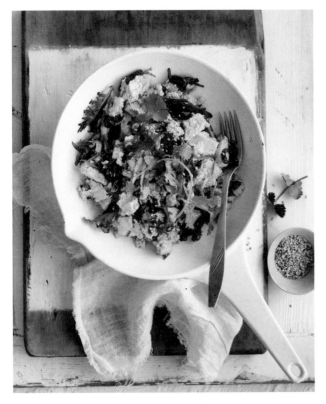
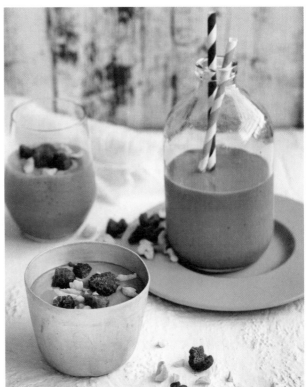
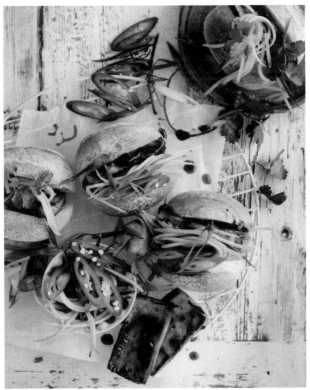
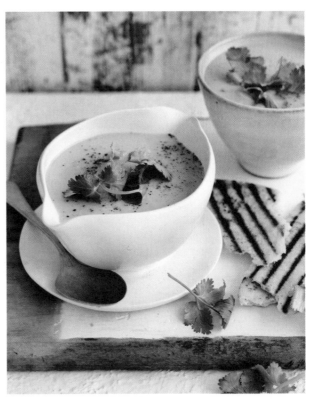

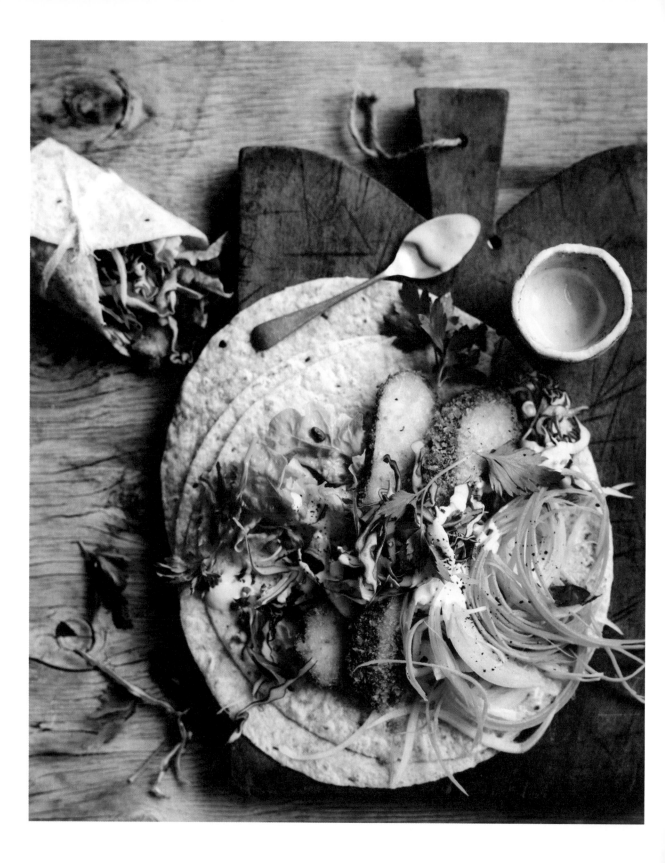

Crumbed courgette and slaw wraps

OVO VEGETARIAN | PREP + COOK TIME **40 MINUTES** | SERVES **4**

Originating in Alabama, white barbecue sauce (also known as Alabama sauce) is a household favourite across the Southern states of the US. Traditionally served as an accompaniment to grilled meat, here it brings a rich and tangy twist to these crunchy veggie wraps.

2 medium courgettes (240g), thinly sliced, lengthways

2 eggs, lightly beaten

1¹/₃ cups (200g) panko breadcrumbs

¹/₄ cup (60ml) olive oil

1 green oak leaf lettuce, leaves separated

4 x 20cm wholegrain wraps (70g)

white barbecue sauce

¹/₄ tsp garlic powder

¹/₄ tsp cayenne pepper

2 tsp horseradish cream

¹/₃ cup (100g) whole-egg mayonnaise

1 tbsp lemon juice

1 tbsp water

slaw

1 cup (80g) finely shredded red cabbage

¹/₂ small white onion (40g), thinly sliced

1 medium carrot (120g), coarsely grated

²/₃ cup (50g) crunchy sprouts, such as sprouted mung beans, adzuki beans, and lentils

salt and freshly ground black pepper

1 To make the white barbecue sauce, stir the ingredients together in a small bowl.

2 To make the slaw, place the cabbage, onion, carrot, sprouts, and half the white barbecue sauce in a medium bowl; toss to combine. Season with salt and pepper to taste

3 Dip the courgette in egg, then coat in the breadcrumbs, pressing lightly to secure.

4 Heat half the olive oil in a large frying pan over a medium-high heat; cook half the courgette for 3 minutes or until both sides are golden and tender. Repeat with the remaining oil and courgette.

5 Place lettuce along the centre of each wrap; top evenly with slaw, courgette, and the remaining white barbecue sauce. Roll to enclose the filling.

Sweet potato and "chorizo" tacos

VEGAN | PREP + COOK TIME **40 MINUTES** | SERVES **4**

These Mexican favourites are often filled with minced beef, but here sweet potato forms the base of a satisfying meat-free "chorizo" that combines sweet and spicy for a tongue-tingling vegan alternative to the traditional taco. Sweet potato can be swapped with pumpkin.

2 small sweet potatoes (500g), unpeeled

$1/2$ cup (120ml) olive oil

6 green onions (spring onions), coarsely chopped

1 tsp ground cumin

1 tsp ground coriander

2 cups (60g) coarsely chopped fresh coriander, roots and stems

2 fresh jalapeño chillies, coarsely chopped

$1^1/2$ tsp finely grated lime rind

2 tbsp lime juice

$1/3$ cup (80ml) water

500g jar sun-dried tomatoes in oil

$1/4$ tsp garlic powder

$1/4$ tsp onion powder

$1/2$ tsp smoked paprika

$1/4$ cup (40g) roasted whole blanched almonds

$1/4$ cup (25g) roasted walnuts

12 x 17cm white corn tortillas, warmed

40g baby rocket leaves

1 Boil, steam, or microwave the sweet potato until tender; drain. When cool enough to handle, peel the sweet potato; cut flesh into 1.5cm pieces.

2 Meanwhile, blend or process the olive oil, onion, cumin, coriander, chillies, lime rind, lime juice, and water in a food processor until smooth. Transfer to a small bowl; stand until required.

3 Drain the oil from the sun-dried tomatoes over a bowl; reserve. Coarsely chop the tomatoes. Process the tomatoes and 2 tablespoons of the reserved oil with the garlic and onion powders, paprika, and nuts until coarsely chopped. Add 2 tablespoons of the coriander mixture; pulse until combined.

4 Transfer the tomato mixture to a large frying pan, stir in the sweet potato. Heat the mixture over a low heat for 5 minutes or until warmed through. Serve the sweet potato mixture in tortillas with rocket and the remaining coriander mixture.

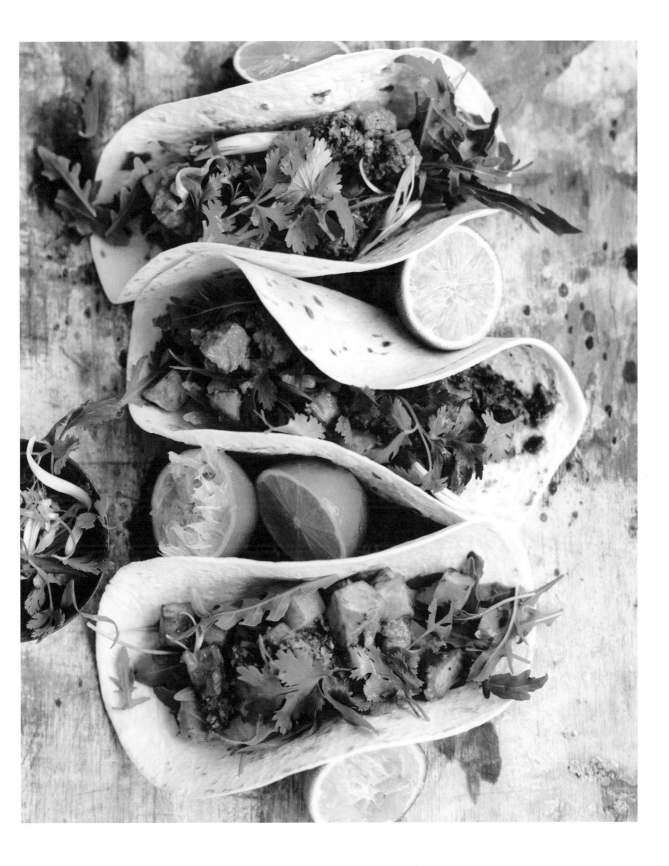

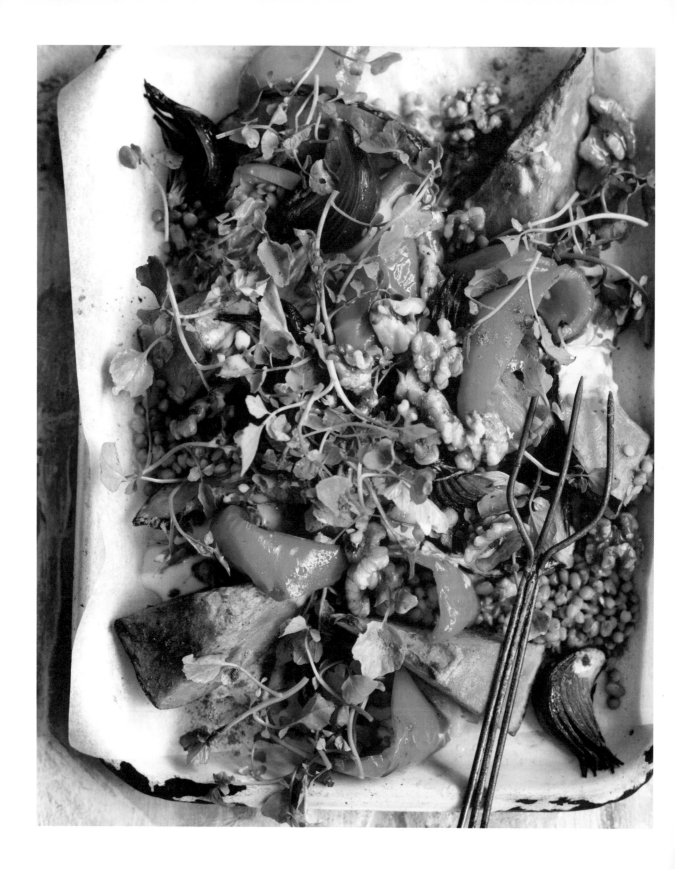

Lebanese roasted pumpkin salad

LACTO VEGETARIAN | PREP + COOK TIME **1 HOUR 15 MINUTES** | SERVES **6**

The Lebanese spices used in this salad lend it Middle Eastern flavours that take it to the next level of salad scrumptiousness. Perfect for a lunch with friends or a light supper. Make extra spice mix and store in an airtight container for up to one month.

2 tbsp honey

1 cup (100g) walnuts

2kg Japanese pumpkin (kabocha squash), cut into 2.5cm thick wedges

1 large red capsicum (pepper) (350g), thickly sliced

1 large red onion (300g), cut into wedges

2 tbsp olive oil

400g can lentils, drained, rinsed

60g watercress

Lebanese spice mix

1 tsp sweet paprika

1 tsp ground cumin

1 tsp ground coriander

1 tsp ground cardamom

$1/2$ tsp ground cinnamon

$1/2$ tsp ground nutmeg

yogurt dressing

$1/2$ cup (140g) Greek yogurt

$1/4$ cup (60ml) olive oil

1 tbsp finely grated lemon rind

$1/4$ cup (60ml) lemon juice

1 tbsp honey

salt and freshly ground black pepper

1 Preheat oven to 200°C (180°C fan/400°F/Gas 6). Line three oven trays with baking paper.

2 To make the Lebanese spice mix, combine ingredients in a small bowl.

3 Bring the honey to the boil in a small frying pan over a medium heat. Add the walnuts and 1 teaspoon of the spice mix; toss gently to coat. Transfer to an oven tray; set aside to cool.

4 Place the pumpkin on another oven tray, and the capsicum and onion on the remaining tray. Drizzle with 2 tablespoons of olive oil and the remaining spice mix; toss to coat. Bake for 30 minutes or until the capsicum and onions are tender; remove from oven.

5 Meanwhile, to make the yogurt dressing, combine the ingredients in a small bowl; season with salt and pepper to taste.

6 Serve the roasted vegetables with the lentils, watercress, nuts, and yogurt dressing.

Vegetable and ginger soba noodle salad

VEGAN | PREP + COOK TIME **30 MINUTES** | SERVES **4**

Wakame has been cultivated in Japan and Korea for use in cuisine for centuries. This bright-green species of edible seaweed is usually sold in dried form, and is perfect for bringing natural umami flavour to soups and salads.

20g wakame (see tips)

200g dried soba noodles

2 cucumbers (260g), seeded, cut into long thin strips

2 small carrots (140g), cut into long thin strips (see tips)

1 fresh long red chilli, seeded, thinly sliced

1 tbsp toasted sesame seeds

3 green onions (spring onions), thinly sliced

1/2 cup (8g) fresh coriander leaves

2cm piece fresh ginger, grated

2 tsp sesame oil

1/4 cup (60ml) lime juice

1 tbsp tamari

1 Place the wakame in a small bowl, cover with cold water; stand for 10 minutes or until the wakame softens. Drain. Discard any hard stems; chop coarsely.

2 Meanwhile, cook the noodles in a small saucepan of boiling water until just tender; drain. Rinse under cold water; drain. Chop noodles coarsely.

3 Place the wakame and noodles in a medium bowl with the remaining ingredients; toss gently to combine. Sprinkle with extra sesame seeds, if you like.

TIPS

- Dried wakame must be softened by soaking for about 10 minutes, and any hard stems are then discarded. It is available from most Asian food stores.
- Use a julienne peeler to cut the cucumber and carrot into long thin strips. Julienne peelers are available from kitchenware stores and some Asian food stores.

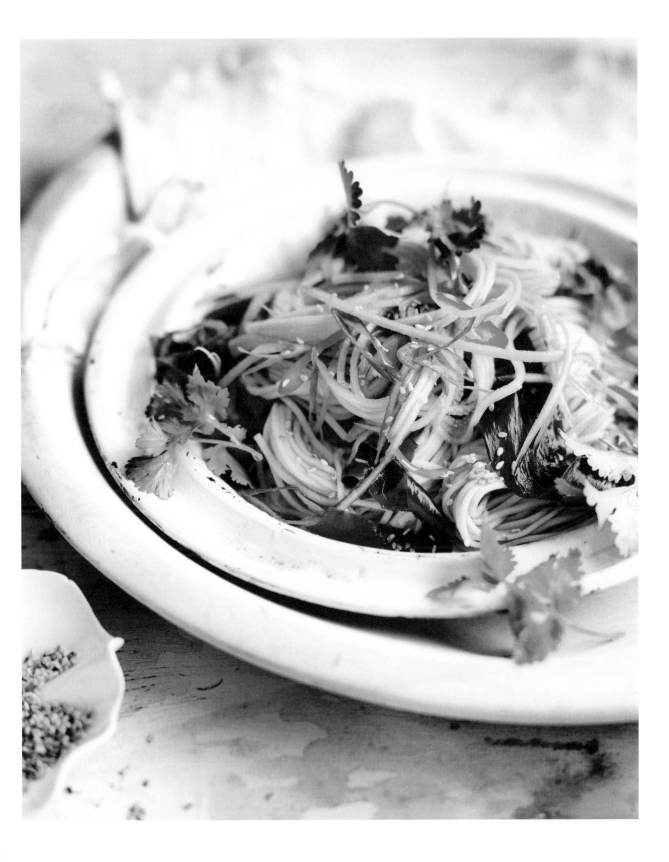

Quinoa, kale, and coriander salad

VEGAN | PREP + COOK TIME **40 MINUTES** | SERVES **4**

Starring two superfoods – kale and quinoa – this dish packs a healthy punch. Naturally low in fat and a great source of protein, tri-colour quinoa brings a nutritious depth to this salad that's delicious enough to stand alone or can be served as a side.

1 cup (200g) tri-colour quinoa

2 cups (500ml) water

450g broccolini (Tenderstem broccoli), trimmed, halved crossways

280g kale, stalks removed, coarsely torn

1/4 cup (50g) pepitas (pumpkin seeds)

1/3 cup (55g) coarsely chopped smoked almonds

2 fresh long green chillies, seeded, thinly sliced

3 garlic cloves, chopped

1/4 cup (60ml) extra virgin olive oil

1 large avocado (320g), chopped

coriander lime dressing

1 cup (16g) fresh coriander leaves

1 fresh long green chilli, seeded, chopped

1/4 cup (60ml) olive oil

2 tbsp lime juice

salt and freshly ground black pepper

1 Preheat oven to 220°C (200°C fan/425°F/Gas 7).

2 Place the quinoa and water in a medium saucepan; bring to the boil. Reduce heat to low; simmer, covered, for 10 minutes or until tender. Rinse under cold water; drain well. Transfer to a large bowl.

3 Combine the broccolini, kale, pepitas, almonds, chilli, garlic, and olive oil in a large shallow baking dish or baking trays; season. Roast for 8 minutes or until the broccolini is tender and the kale is wilted, stirring twice during cooking.

4 Meanwhile, to make the coriander lime dressing, place the ingredients in a blender or food processor; pulse until finely chopped. Season with salt and pepper to taste.

5 Add the kale mixture to the quinoa; toss gently to combine. Serve the salad topped with avocado and drizzled with dressing.

TIPS

- Cauliflower is also delicious roasted in the same way; allow an extra 10 minutes cooking time.
- Squeeze a little extra lime juice over the avocado to prevent browning if you are packaging and transporting the salad.

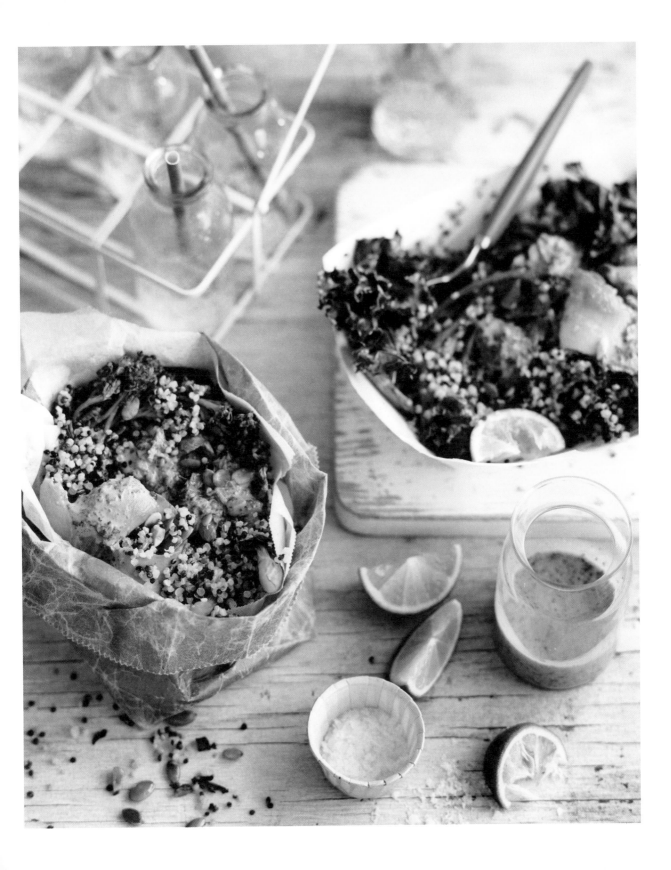

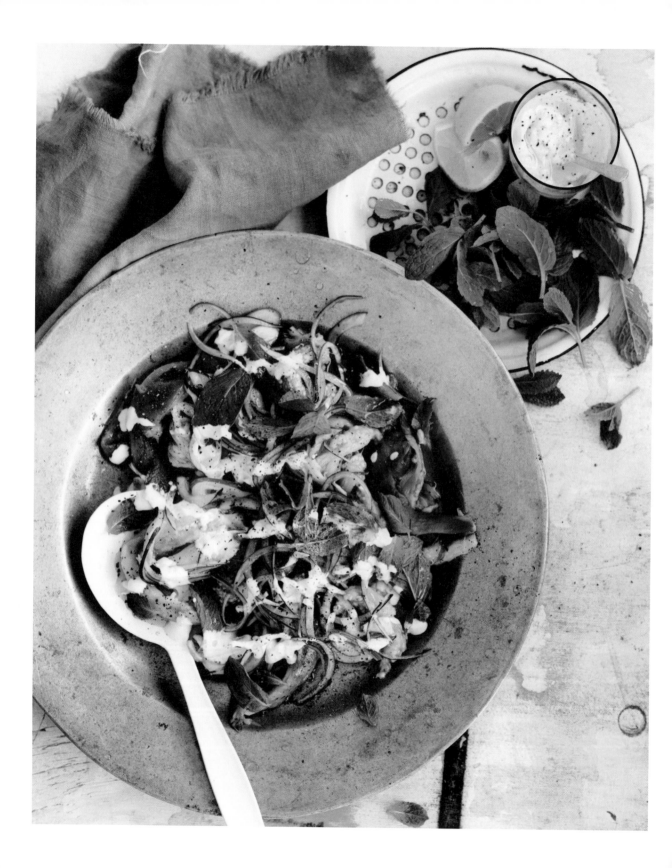

Smoky aubergine salad with tahini

LACTO VEGETARIAN | PREP + COOK TIME **45 MINUTES** | SERVES **8**

This recipe is perfect for a light lunch, a summer picnic, or to serve as part of a mezze banquet. Transport the aubergine salad and yogurt sauce separately. Assemble the salad just before serving.

1 small red onion (100g), halved, very thinly sliced

2 tbsp lemon juice

5 medium aubergines (1.5kg)

1½ tbsp tahini

2 garlic cloves, crushed

1 cup (280g) Greek yogurt

salt and freshly ground black pepper

2 tbsp extra virgin olive oil

1 cup (8g) fresh mint leaves, extra, torn

1 tsp sumac

1 Combine the onion and half the lemon juice in a small bowl; set aside.

2 Preheat a barbecue or char-grill plate to a high heat. Prick the aubergines all over with a fork. Cook the aubergines on the heated barbecue, turning occasionally, for 30 minutes or until the skin is charred and the flesh is very tender. Place the aubergines in a large sieve over a large bowl; drain. Cool.

3 Meanwhile, combine the tahini, garlic, yogurt, and remaining lemon juice in a small bowl. Season with salt and pepper to taste.

4 Remove and discard the skin from the aubergines. Using two forks, pull apart the flesh into pieces. Spoon the aubergine onto a large serving platter; season well with salt and pepper, then drizzle with olive oil. Serve topped with the onion mixture, mint, and yogurt sauce. Sprinkle with sumac.

Za'atar chickpeas and vegetable salad

LACTO VEGETARIAN | PREP + COOK TIME **45 MINUTES** | SERVES **4**

When roasting the vegetables, ensure they are placed in a single layer on the oven tray so they roast quickly without steaming. If necessary, divide the vegetables between two trays. Serve with grilled flatbread.

400g butternut pumpkin (butternut squash), unpeeled

1 large red onion (300g), cut into thin wedges

1 medium red capsicum (pepper) (200g), thickly sliced

1 medium yellow capsicum (pepper) (200g), thickly sliced

400g baby rainbow carrots, trimmed

2 tbsp olive oil

salt and freshly ground black pepper

400g can chickpeas, drained, rinsed

2 tbsp za'atar

$1/4$ cup (60ml) red wine vinegar

$1/4$ cup (60ml) olive oil, extra

60g red veined sorrel or baby spinach leaves

100g Persian feta, crumbled

$1/3$ cup (3g) small fresh mint leaves

1 Preheat oven to 220°C (200°C fan/425°F/Gas 7). Line a large oven tray with baking paper.

2 Cut the unpeeled pumpkin into thin wedges; halve crossways. Place the pumpkin, onion, capsicums, and carrots, in a single layer, on the oven tray; drizzle with half the olive oil, then season with salt and pepper. Bake for 25 minutes or until tender.

3 Meanwhile, place the chickpeas on another baking-paper-lined oven tray. Drizzle with the remaining olive oil, sprinkle with za'atar; toss gently to coat. Bake for 25 minutes or until golden and crisp.

4 Whisk the vinegar and extra olive oil in a small bowl; season with salt and pepper.

5 Pour the dressing into two 2-cup (500ml) jars. Layer all the ingredients in the jars finishing with the feta and chickpeas.

TIPS

- Baby rainbow carrots are also sold as heirloom carrots; they are available from some supermarkets and greengrocers.
- This salad makes a great portable lunch – simply secure the lid to seal the jar and off you go. When you're ready to serve, turn the lidded jars upside down to disperse the dressing.

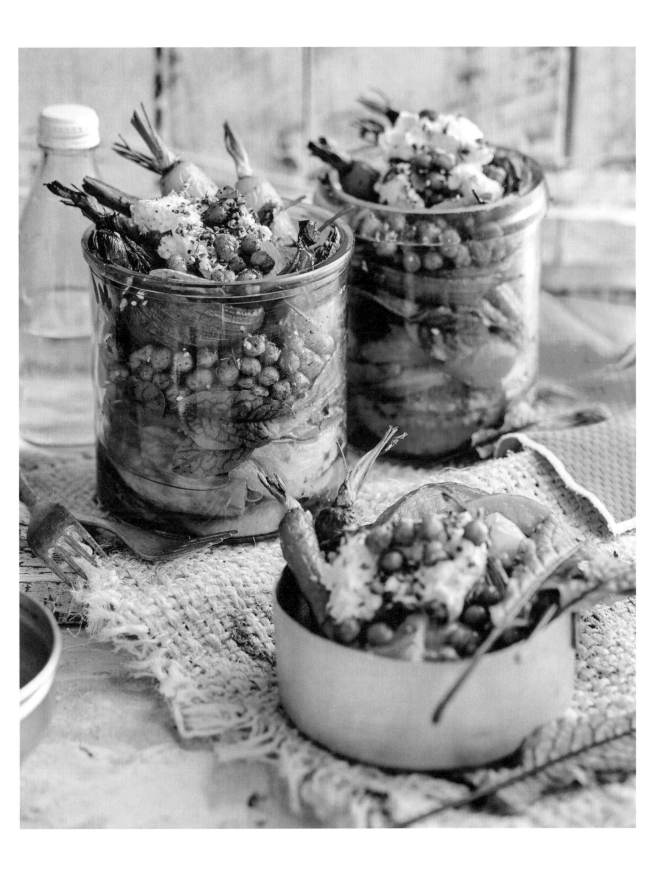

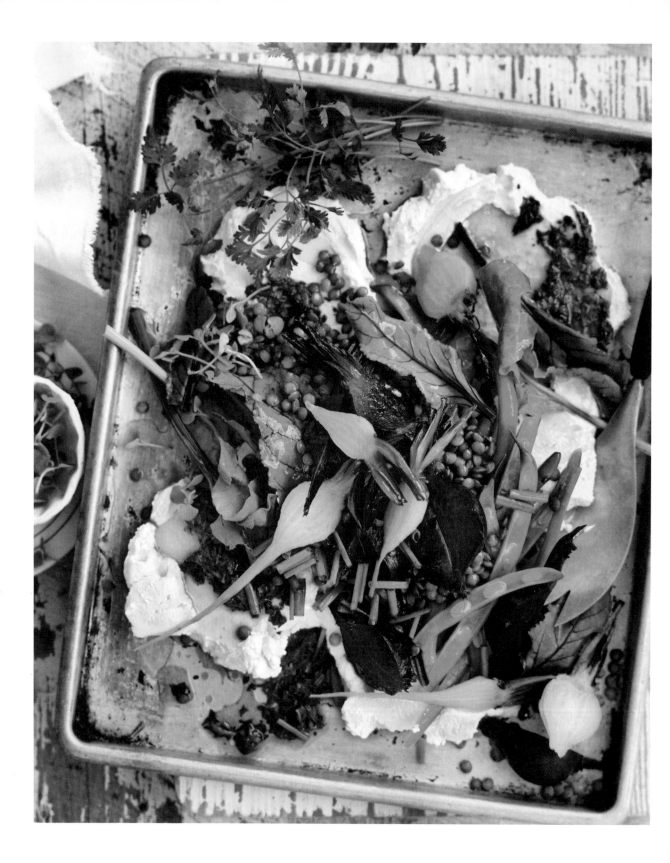

Lentil, beetroot, and labneh salad

LACTO VEGETARIAN | PREP + COOK TIME **1 HOUR 15 MINUTES + REFRIGERATION** | SERVES **6**

Labneh is a type of soft cheese popular in Middle Eastern cuisine. It is made by straining Greek yogurt until it loses most of its liquid. The creamy labneh perfectly offsets the earthy beetroot in this showstopping salad. You need to start this recipe a day ahead.

1kg Greek yogurt

500g baby beetroot, trimmed, small leaves reserved

500g golden baby beetroot, trimmed, small leaves reserved

2 tbsp olive oil

1 cup (200g) green lentils

120g baby spinach leaves

2 tbsp lemon juice

¼ cup (60ml) olive oil, extra

salt and freshly ground black pepper

150g baby green beans, trimmed

½ cup (10g) loosely packed fresh baby basil leaves

½ cup (30g) fresh flat-leaf parsley leaves

½ cup (4g) fresh chervil leaves

½ cup (30g) finely chopped fresh chives

dressing

2 tbsp olive oil

2 tbsp red wine vinegar

1 tsp sugar

TIPS

- If you don't have time to make your own labneh, you can use 3 cups (840g) store-bought labneh.
- Use mixed salad leaves if no beetroot leaves are available.
- The dressing can be made 1 week ahead; refrigerate in the jar.

1 To make the labneh, line a large sieve with two layers of muslin or cheesecloth; place the sieve over a deep bowl or jug large enough to hold the sieve. Spoon the yogurt into the sieve, gather the cloth and tie into a ball with kitchen string. Hang above the bowl. Refrigerate for 24 hours or until thick, gently squeezing occasionally to encourage the liquid to drain. Discard liquid. Transfer labneh to a large bowl.

2 Preheat oven to 180°C (160°C fan/350°F/Gas 4).

3 Trim the beetroot; reserve 100g of the smallest beetroot leaves. Wash the beetroot well. Place in a roasting pan; drizzle with olive oil. Cover the pan with foil; roast for 45 minutes or until tender. Stand for 10 minutes. When cool enough to handle, remove the skins (they should slip off easily; if not use a small knife). Cut the beetroot into halves or quarters.

4 Meanwhile, cook the lentils in a medium saucepan of boiling water, for 12 minutes or until tender; drain. Rinse under cold water; drain well.

5 Blend or process the spinach, lemon juice, and extra olive oil until well combined. Season with salt and pepper to taste.

6 Pour boiling water over the beans in a large heatproof bowl; stand for 1 minute. Drain. Refresh the beans in another bowl of iced water; drain well.

7 To make the dressing, place the ingredients in a screw-top jar; shake well. Season with salt and pepper to taste.

8 Place the beetroot, lentils, and beans in a large bowl with the herbs, reserved beetroot leaves, and half the dressing; toss gently to combine.

9 Spread the labneh on a serving tray; top with the spinach mixture and salad. Drizzle with the remaining dressing.

Smoked tofu salad with peanut dressing

OVO VEGETARIAN | PREP + COOK TIME **45 MINUTES** | SERVES **4**

Smoked tofu is most often smoked in tea leaves, giving it an attractive light hue and a distinctive taste. It's great to use in any dish where you're wanting a smoky flavour and a chewy texture. It pairs beautifully with a spiced nutty dressing such as this.

4 eggs

1/4 cup (60ml) water

1 tbsp fried Asian shallots

1 tsp tamari

salt and freshly ground black pepper

1 tbsp sesame oil

350g smoked tofu, cut into 1cm pieces

1 medium avocado (250g), thinly sliced

250g cherry tomatoes, halved

1 1/2 cups (120g) bean sprouts

1/2 cup (8g) fresh coriander leaves

1/2 cup (4g) fresh vietnamese mint leaves

75g baby salad leaves

2 tbsp black sesame seeds

peanut dressing

1/3 cup (45g) roasted peanuts, coarsely chopped

1 green onion (spring onion), thinly sliced

1 fresh long red chilli, thinly sliced

1 tsp finely grated fresh ginger

1 garlic clove, crushed

1 1/2 tbsp grated palm sugar

2 tbsp sesame oil

2 tbsp tamari

1/4 cup (60ml) rice vinegar

1 1/2 tbsp lime juice

1 To make the peanut dressing, whisk the ingredients in a medium bowl until combined.

2 Whisk the eggs, water, shallots, and tamari in a large bowl; season with salt and pepper.

3 Heat the sesame oil in a wok over a medium heat. Pour half the egg mixture into the wok; cook, tilting the wok, until almost set. Remove the omelette from the wok. Repeat with the remaining egg mixture. Roll omelettes tightly, then slice thinly; reserve.

4 Place the tofu in a large bowl with the remaining ingredients and peanut dressing; toss to combine.

5 Serve the tofu salad topped with the reserved omelette.

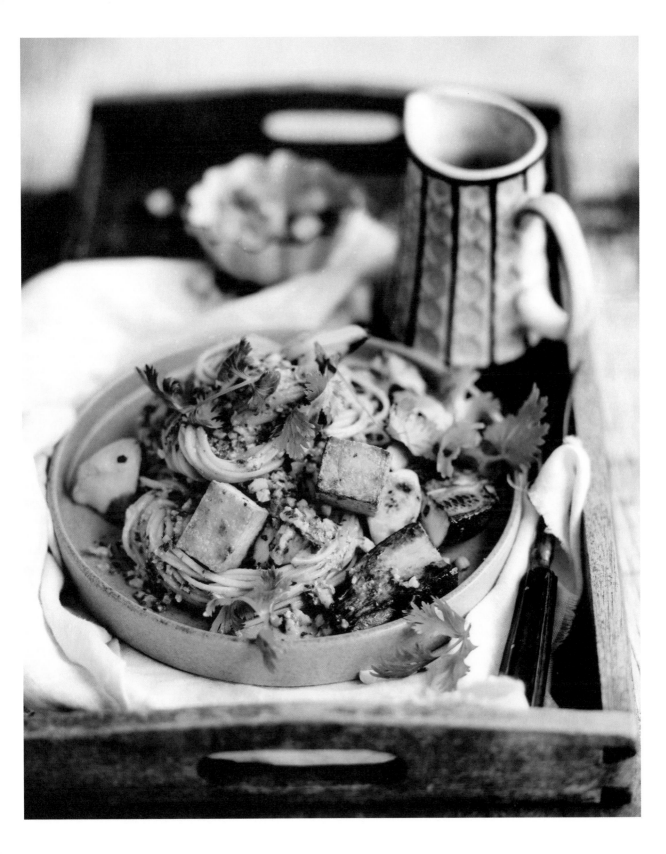

Miso vegetables with pounded rice salad

VEGAN | PREP + COOK TIME **30 MINUTES** | SERVES **4**

White miso (shiro) is a fermented bean paste that lies at the heart of Japanese cuisine. Made from soybeans and rice it contains millions of beneficial bacteria essential to good gut health. Here it brings an umami depth to this perfectly balanced sauce.

2 tbsp sesame oil

4 king brown mushrooms (king oyster mushrooms), trimmed, quartered lengthways

170g asparagus, trimmed, halved lengthways

6 green onions (spring onions), trimmed, thinly sliced

400g enoki mushrooms, trimmed

pounded rice salad

¼ cup (55g) sushi rice

1 large (350g) yellow capsicum (pepper), finely sliced

1 large (350g) red capsicum (pepper), finely sliced

½ cup (10g) loosely packed coriander leaves

½ cup (4g) loosely packed vietnamese mint leaves

1 cup (100g) bean sprouts

2 tbsp sesame seeds, toasted

miso sauce

¼ cup (60g) white (shiro) miso

¼ cup (60ml) rice vinegar

1 tbsp pure maple syrup

1 tsp finely chopped pickled ginger

1 tbsp pickled ginger juice

½ tsp dried chilli flakes

salt and freshly ground black pepper

1 To make the pounded rice salad, heat a large frying pan over a medium heat, add the rice; stir continuously for 4 minutes or until the rice is lightly golden and toasted. Grind the toasted rice with a mortar and pestle to a fine powder. Place the ground rice in a medium bowl with the remaining ingredients; toss to combine.

2 To make the miso sauce, whisk the ingredients together in a small bowl; season with salt and pepper.

3 Heat a wok over a medium high heat. Add the sesame oil and king brown mushrooms; stir-fry for 5 minutes. Transfer to a tray. Stir-fry the asparagus and green onions for 2 minutes; transfer to the tray. Stir-fry the enoki mushrooms for 30 seconds or until heated through; transfer to the tray.

4 Serve the vegetables topped with the miso sauce and the rice salad.

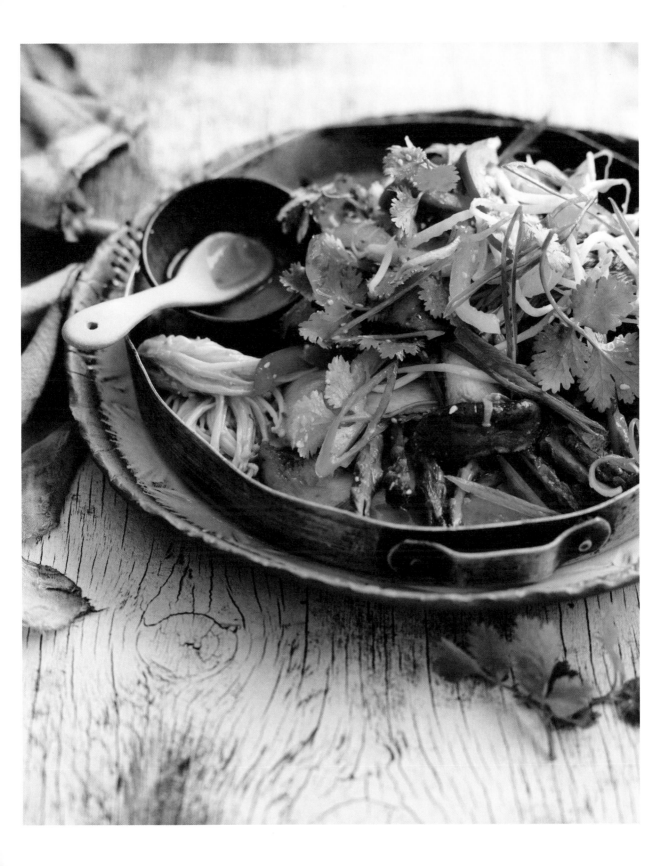

Pear and walnut salad with tarragon pesto

LACTO VEGETARIAN | PREP + COOK TIME **30 MINUTES** | SERVES **4**

Although more commonly made with basil, tarragon makes for a flavourful twist on a classic pesto. Using good quality olive oil will help give your tarragon pesto a deep and rich flavour. Bold and aromatic, it's the ideal companion to the sweet pear and walnuts.

4 small corella pears (400g), thickly sliced crossways

2 stalks celery (300g), trimmed, sliced diagonally (see tips)

1 cup (15g) firmly packed fresh celery leaves

1 baby fennel (130g), very thinly sliced (see tips)

1/2 cup (50g) walnuts, roasted, coarsely chopped

salt and freshly ground black pepper

100g blue cheese, coarsely crumbled

tarragon pesto

1 cup (24g) fresh tarragon leaves

2 slices white bread (90g), crusts removed

1/4 cup (60ml) milk

1/4 cup (60ml) water

2 tbsp olive oil

1 tsp sea salt

1 To make the tarragon pesto, blend or process the ingredients until well combined.

2 Cook the pear on a heated oiled barbecue (or grill or grill pan) until lightly browned on both sides.

3 Place the pear in a large bowl with the celery and celery leaves, fennel, and walnuts; toss gently to combine. Season with salt and pepper to taste.

4 Serve the salad topped with the pesto and blue cheese.

TIPS

- Use the yellow and lighter green leaves from the heart of the celery.
- Use a mandoline or V-slicer to cut the fennel into very thin slices.

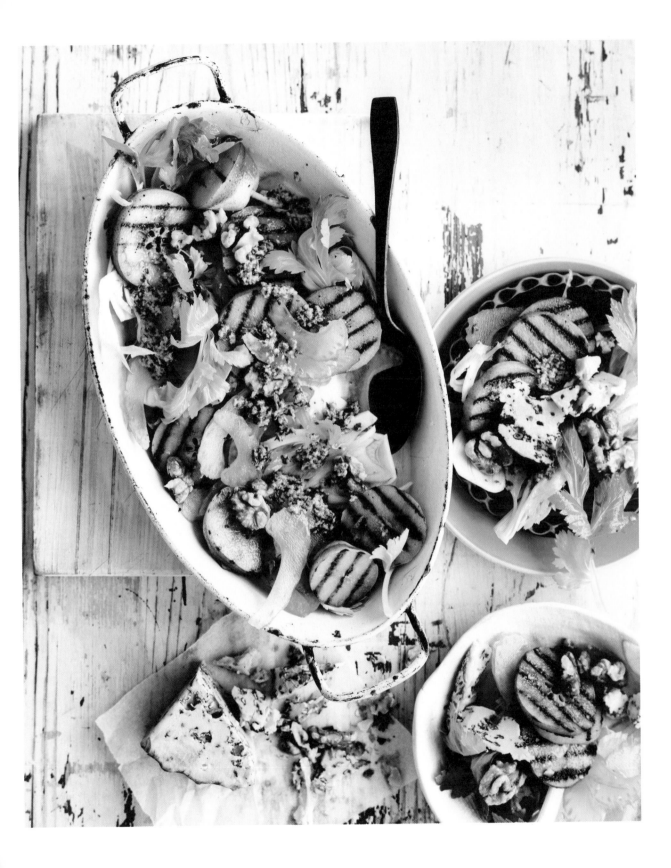

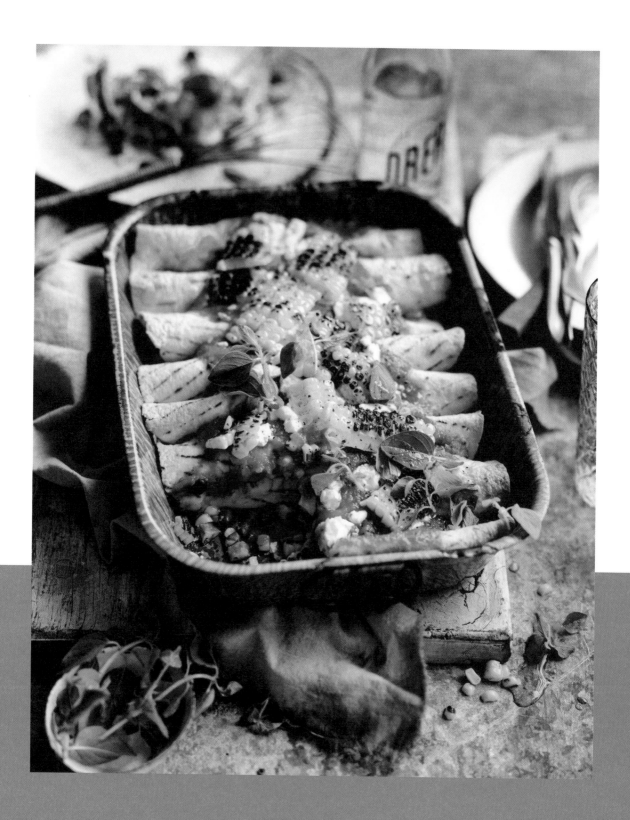

HEARTY MAINS

These comfort food classics with a veggie twist will keep you warm and toasty on a winter's night. Tuck into tasty stews, curries, soups, and pasta bakes.

Sweet potato cannelloni

OVO VEGETARIAN | PREP + COOK TIME **1 HOUR 15 MINUTES** | SERVES **6**

Thinly sliced sweet potato replaces pasta in this veggie take on an Italian classic. If you prefer, you could layer the sweet potato slices and filling mixture instead of rolling them. Leftover sweet potato can be chopped and cooked in soups, purees, and mashes.

3 medium sweet potatoes (1.2kg), unpeeled

500g fresh ricotta

1 egg, lightly beaten

2 green onions (spring onions), thinly sliced

$1/4$ cup (6g) finely chopped fresh flat-leaf parsley

$1/4$ cup (15g) finely chopped fresh chives

2 tbsp finely chopped fresh thyme

1 cup (80g) finely grated vegetarian parmesan (make sure it doesn't contain animal rennet)

1 cup (80g) finely grated pecorino cheese

100g sourdough bread, crust removed, torn into small pieces

$1/4$ cup (40g) pine nuts

$1/2$ tsp ground nutmeg

$1^{1}/_{2}$ tbsp olive oil

$1/3$ cup (25g) shaved vegetarian parmesan, extra

2 tbsp fresh thyme sprigs, extra

salt and freshly ground black pepper

cheese sauce

1 cup (250ml) thickened (double) cream

$3/4$ cup (90g) coarsely grated vegetarian cheddar

1 Preheat oven to 200°C (180°C fan/400°F/Gas 6). Place one of the sweet potatoes on an oven tray. Bake for 30 minutes or until tender; cool. Reduce oven to 160°C (140°C fan/325°F/Gas 3).

2 Meanwhile, peel the remaining sweet potatoes. Using a mandoline or V-slicer, cut the sweet potatoes lengthways into 3mm thin slices. Trim the slices to 5.5cm x 12cm rectangles; you will need 36 rectangles.

3 Bring a large saucepan of water to the boil. Add half the sweet potato slices; boil for $1^{1}/_{2}$ minutes or until softened. Remove from the pan with a slotted spoon; place on a tray to cool. Repeat with the remaining sweet potato slices.

4 When cool enough to handle, remove the skin from the baked sweet potato. Add the baked sweet potato to a processor with the ricotta; process until smooth. Transfer to a large bowl. Stir in the egg, green onion, herbs, and half the cheeses. Season with salt and pepper.

5 Oil a 22cm x 26cm roasting pan. Place a heaped tablespoon of filling at the short end of a sweet potato slice; roll to enclose the filling. Place, seam-side down, in the pan. Repeat with the remaining sweet potato slices and filling, until the pan is filled, in a single layer.

6 Combine the sourdough, pine nuts, and nutmeg in a medium bowl with 1 tablespoon of the olive oil and the remaining cheeses. Sprinkle over the sweet potato cannelloni.

7 Bake for 15 minutes or until the top is golden and crunchy.

8 Meanwhile, to make the cheese sauce, stir the ingredients in a small saucepan over a medium heat, without boiling, for 4 minutes or until the cheddar melts and sauce thickens slightly. Season with salt and pepper.

9 Serve the sweet potato cannelloni topped with the cheese sauce, extra shaved vegetarian parmesan, and extra thyme; drizzle with the remaining olive oil.

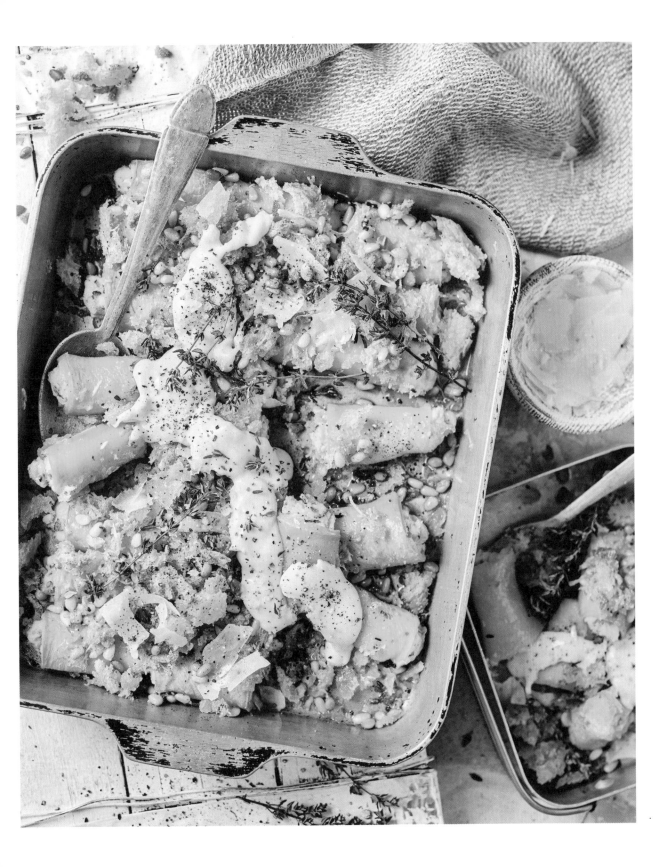

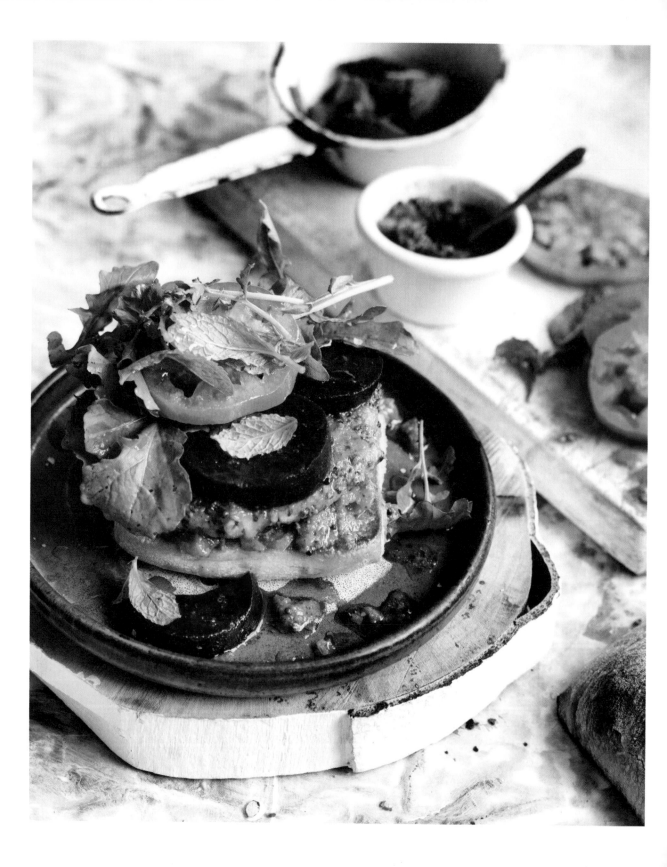

Quinoa, courgette, and haloumi burger

LACTO-OVO VEGETARIAN | PREP + COOK TIME **45 MINUTES + REFRIGERATION** | SERVES **6**

This is a great dish for when you're entertaining or if you're short on time as the patties can be prepared a day ahead and kept, covered, in the refrigerator. They can then be cooked and the burgers assembled when you're ready to eat.

½ cup (100g) red quinoa

1 cup (250ml) water

1 large courgette (150g), coarsely grated

250g haloumi, coarsely grated

⅓ cup (16g) finely chopped fresh mint

⅓ cup (20g) finely chopped fresh chives

2 eggs, lightly beaten

1 cup (120g) plain flour

salt and freshly ground black pepper

1 tbsp olive oil

6 sourdough rolls (550g), halved, toasted

⅓ cup (95g) tomato kasundi or chutney

200g vacuum-packed cooked beetroot, sliced

300g heirloom tomatoes, sliced

60g baby rocket leaves

½ cup (4g) fresh mint leaves, extra

1 Place the quinoa and the water in a small saucepan; bring to the boil. Reduce heat to low; simmer gently, for 15 minutes or until most of the water is absorbed. Remove from heat; cover, stand for 5 minutes. Transfer to a large bowl; cool.

2 Add the courgette to the quinoa with the haloumi, chopped mint, chives, egg, and ⅔ cup (85g) of the flour; season with salt and pepper, then mix well. Shape the mixture into six patties with damp hands. Place on a plate; refrigerate for 30 minutes.

3 When ready to fry, coat the patties in the remaining flour. Heat the olive oil in a medium non-stick frying pan over a medium heat; cook the patties for 4 minutes each side or until golden brown.

4 Preheat your oven to 180°C (350°F). Slice each ciabatta roll in half and brush the insides with 1 tbsp of olive oil. Toast for 5 minutes or until golden brown.

5 To assemble, top the base of the rolls with kasundi, patties, beetroot, tomato, rocket, and extra mint. Top with the bread roll tops.

Spiced lentil and sweet potato pies

LACTO-OVO VEGETARIAN | PREP + COOK TIME **1 HOUR 20 MINUTES + COOLING** | MAKES **8**

Harissa tends to be a hot chilli paste; there are many different brands available on the market, and the strengths vary enormously. If you have a low heat-level tolerance, use a milder chilli paste instead.

2 tbsp olive oil

1 medium red onion (170g), finely chopped

3 garlic cloves, finely chopped

1 celery stalk (150g), trimmed, finely chopped

2 tbsp harissa

1 tsp ground cumin

1 tsp ground coriander

2^1/$_4$ cups (450g) green lentils

2 small sweet potatoes (500g), cut into 3cm pieces

2 cups (500ml) vegetable stock

^{1}/$_2$ cup (125ml) water

400g can cherry tomatoes in juice

60g baby spinach leaves

^{1}/$_2$ cup (30g) fresh flat-leaf parsley leaves

^{1}/$_2$ cup (8g) fresh coriander leaves

1^1/$_2$ tsp finely grated lemon rind

salt and freshly ground black pepper

4 sheets puff pastry

1 free-range egg, lightly beaten

herb and lemon yogurt

1 cup (280g) Greek yogurt

^{1}/$_4$ cup (5g) coarsely chopped fresh flat-leaf parsley

^{1}/$_4$ cup (8g) coarsely chopped fresh coriander

1 tbsp finely chopped preserved lemon rind

1 tbsp lemon juice

1 Heat the olive oil in a large saucepan over a medium heat; cook the onion, garlic, and celery for 5 minutes or until the onion softens. Add the harissa and spices, cook, stirring, for 1 minute or until fragrant. Add the lentils, sweet potato, stock, and the water; bring to the boil. Reduce heat, simmer, covered, for 20 minutes or until the lentils and sweet potato are tender.

2 Add the tomatoes; return to a simmer, cook, uncovered, for 5 minutes or until thickened. Stir in the spinach, parsley, fresh coriander, and lemon rind; season with salt and pepper to taste; cool.

3 Meanwhile, to make the herb and lemon yogurt, combine the ingredients in a bowl.

4 Preheat oven to 200°C (180°C fan/400°F/Gas 6). Grease eight 1-cup (250ml) pie tins (with a base measurement of 7.5cm and a top measurement of 12.5cm).

5 Cut eight 13cm squares from the pastry. Refrigerate until required.

6 Fill the pie tins with cooled lentil filling; top with the pastry squares, pressing the edges to seal. Brush the tops with egg. Cut small steam holes in the top of the pies.

7 Bake the pies for 30 minutes or until the pastry is golden and the filling is hot. Serve with the herb and lemon yogurt.

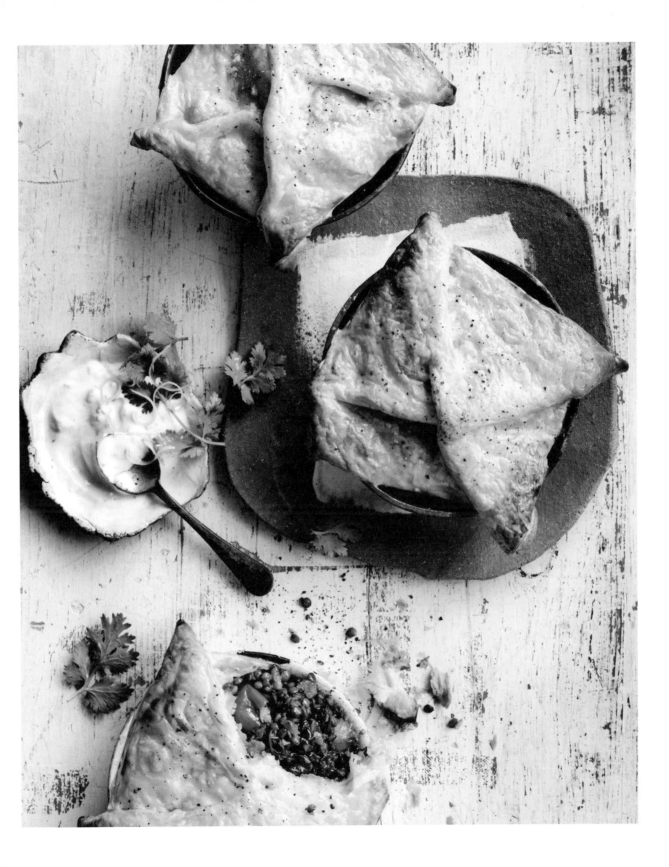

Soft polenta with mushroom ragu

LACTO VEGETARIAN | PREP + COOK TIME **30 MINUTES** | SERVES **4**

You could also top the polenta with ratatouille or a selection of mixed roasted
vegetables such as pumpkin, onion, capsicum, aubergine, and courgette.
Serve with a fresh mixed herb salad.

30g butter

500g cup mushrooms, thickly sliced

3 garlic cloves, crushed

1/2 cup (125ml) vegetable stock

salt and freshly ground black pepper

150g soft goat's cheese

1/4 cup (15g) fresh flat-leaf parsley leaves

soft polenta

2 cups (500ml) milk

2 cups (500ml) vegetable stock

1 cup (170g) instant polenta

40g butter, chopped

3/4 cup (60g) finely grated vegetarian parmesan

1 Heat the butter in a large frying pan over a high heat; cook the mushrooms, stirring occasionally, for 5 minutes or until the mushrooms are lightly browned and most of the liquid has evaporated. Add the garlic; cook, stirring, until fragrant. Stir in the stock; bring to the boil. Reduce the heat; simmer, for 2 minutes or until most of the liquid has evaporated. Season with salt and pepper to taste; cover to keep warm.

2 Meanwhile, to make the soft polenta, bring the milk and stock to the boil in a large saucepan. Gradually add the polenta, stirring constantly. Reduce heat; cook, stirring frequently, for 10 minutes or until the polenta thickens. Stir in the butter and vegetarian parmesan. Season with salt and pepper to taste.

3 Pour the polenta immediately onto a serving board or plate; using the back of a spoon, make slight hollows in the polenta. Spoon the mushrooms over the polenta using a slotted spoon; drizzle with some of the pan juices. Top with small chunks of the goat's cheese; sprinkle with parsley.

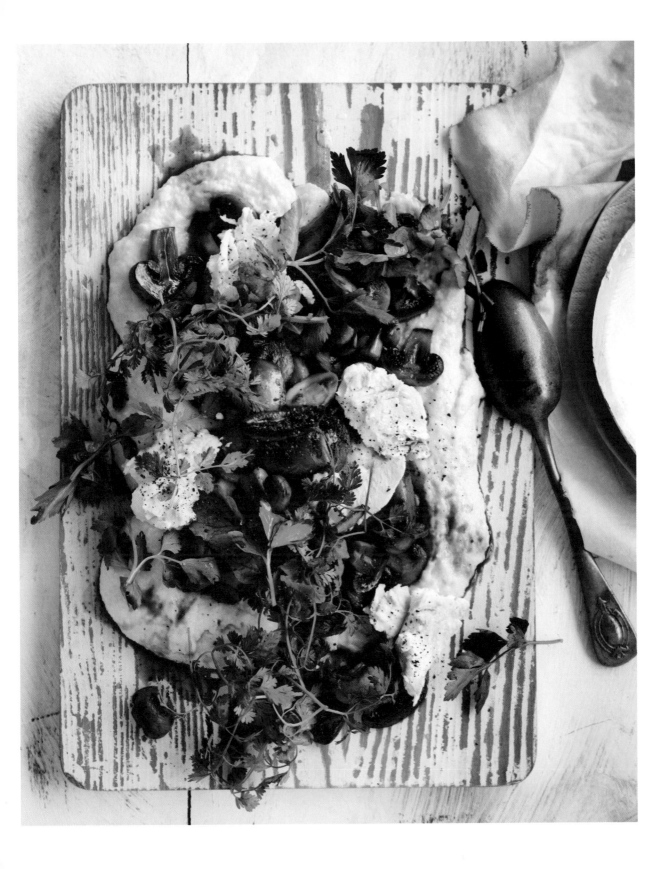

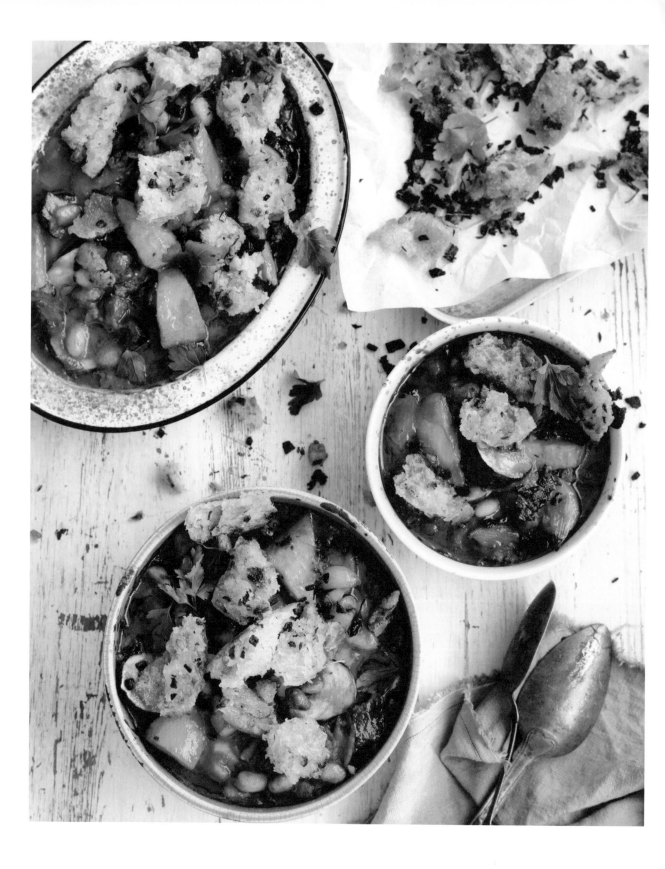

Vegetable cassoulet

VEGAN | PREP + COOK TIME **1 HOUR 15 MINUTES + STANDING** | SERVES **4**

Originating in Languedoc in Southwest France, cassoulet takes its name from its cooking pot, the cassole d'Issel. Rich and slow-cooked, this vegan twist on the French classic is full of hearty flavours that mirror its meaty counterpart. Serve with a bitter leaf salad.

2 tsp olive oil

4 shallots (100g), halved

3 garlic cloves, thinly sliced

2 medium carrots (240g), coarsely chopped

200g swiss brown mushrooms (chestnut mushrooms), halved

1 cup (250ml) dry white wine

2 medium courgettes (240g), coarsely chopped

1½ cups (375ml) vegetable stock

700g bottled tomato puree (passata)

1 tsp finely chopped fresh thyme

400g can borlotti beans, drained, rinsed

bread topping

1 tbsp olive oil

1 small brown onion (80g), finely chopped

1 garlic clove, crushed

2 tsp finely grated lemon rind

2 tsp finely chopped fresh thyme

½ wholegrain and seed sourdough bread (220g), torn into 2cm pieces

2 tbsp coarsely chopped fresh flat-leaf parsley

1 Preheat oven to 180°C (160°C fan/350°F/Gas 4).

2 Heat the olive oil in a large flameproof casserole dish over a medium-high heat; cook the shallot, garlic, carrot, and mushrooms, stirring, for 5 minutes or until the vegetables are just tender. Add the wine; bring to the boil. Boil until the liquid is reduced by half. Add the courgette, stock, tomato puree, thyme, and beans; return to the boil. Remove from the heat. Cover dish; transfer to the oven, cook for 50 minutes.

3 Meanwhile, to make the bread topping, heat the olive oil in a large frying pan over a medium-high heat; cook the onion, stirring, for 5 minutes or until soft. Add the garlic, lemon rind, thyme, and bread; cook, stirring, for 10 minutes or until the bread lightly browns. Stir in the parsley.

4 Season the cassoulet to taste, sprinkle with bread topping; return to the oven, uncovered, for 10 minutes or until the bread topping is browned.

Courgette, black bean, and corn enchiladas

LACTO VEGETARIAN | PREP + COOK TIME **1 HOUR 40 MINUTES** | SERVES **4**

Enchiladas featured in one of the first-ever Mexican cookbooks in the early 1800s. Still a Mexican favourite, this is a versatile dish that can be adapted to suit everyone's tastes. Here the traditional meat filling is replaced with protein-rich black beans.

3 large courgettes (450g)

⅓ cup (80ml) olive oil

2 trimmed corn cobs (500g)

8 x 20cm white corn tortillas

400g can black beans, drained, rinsed

½ cup (8g) fresh coriander leaves

100g feta

¼ cup (3g) fresh oregano leaves

1 tbsp fresh oregano, extra

enchilada sauce

2 x 400g can chopped tomatoes

1½ cups (375ml) vegetable stock

2 tbsp olive oil

2 tbsp coarsely chopped fresh oregano

2 tbsp apple cider vinegar

1 medium brown onion (150g), coarsely chopped

1 garlic clove, chopped

1 tbsp chopped pickled jalapeños

1 tsp ground cumin

1 tsp caster sugar

¼ tsp ground chilli powder

1 Preheat oven to 180°C (160°C fan/350°F/Gas 4). Line an oven tray with baking paper. Grease a 25cm x 30cm ovenproof dish.

2 Cut the courgettes in half lengthways then cut each half into long thin wedges. Place the courgette on the oven tray; drizzle with half the olive oil. Roast for 30 minutes or until just tender; chop coarsely.

3 Meanwhile to make the enchilada sauce, blend or process the ingredients until smooth; transfer to a medium saucepan. Bring to a simmer over a medium heat for 20 minutes or until thickened slightly.

4 Brush the corn with 1 tablespoon of the olive oil. Heat a grill plate (or grill or barbecue) over a medium-high heat; cook the corn, turning occasionally, for 10 minutes or until golden and tender. Using a sharp knife, cut the kernels from the cobs; discard cobs.

5 Reheat the grill plate (or grill or barbecue) over a medium-high heat; cook the tortillas, for 30 seconds each side or until lightly charred. Transfer to a plate; cover to keep warm.

6 Combine the courgette, beans, coriander, half the corn, half the feta, half the oregano, and ½ cup (225g) of enchilada sauce in a large bowl.

7 Divide the courgette filling evenly among the warm tortillas; roll to enclose the filling. Place the tortillas in a dish; brush the tops with the remaining olive oil. Spoon the remaining enchilada sauce over the tortillas, leaving 2cm at each end of the enchiladas uncovered. Top with the remaining feta and oregano.

8 Bake for 30 minutes or until golden and heated through. Serve topped with the remaining corn and extra oregano.

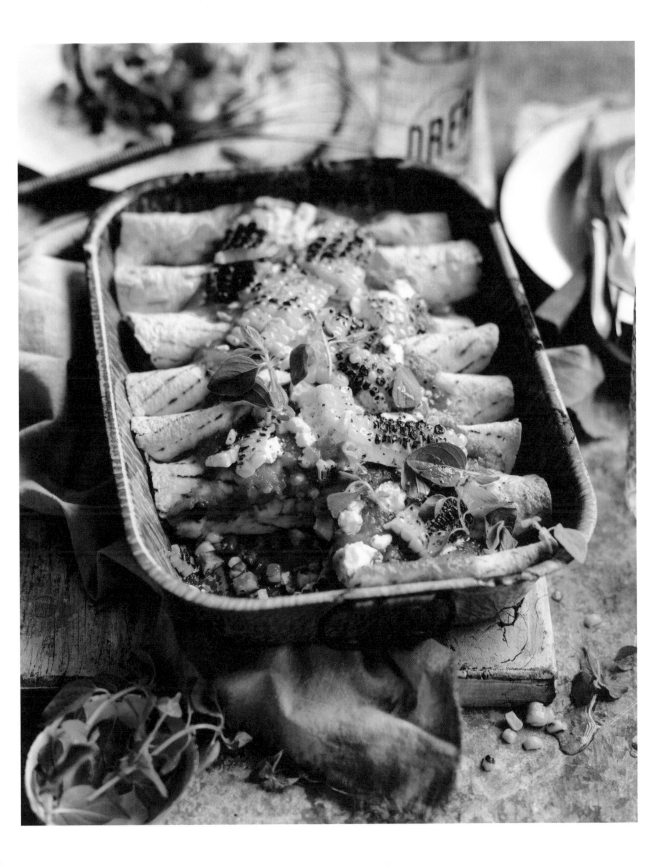

Broccoli pizza with courgette

LACTO-OVO VEGETARIAN | PREP + COOK TIME **1 HOUR 15 MINUTES** | SERVES **4**

This healthy low carb broccoli base provides a nutritious and flavourful alternative to pizza dough. You can use your favourite pasta sauce in place of the tomato puree (passata), if you like and top with vegetables of your choice.

1kg broccoli, trimmed, cut into florets

¼ cup (30g) coarsely grated vegetarian cheddar

1 egg, lightly beaten

¾ cup (60g) coarsely grated vegetarian parmesan (make sure it doesn't contain animal rennet)

salt and freshly ground black pepper

½ cup (130g) tomato puree (passata)

2 small courgettes (180g), thinly sliced into ribbons

1 cup (20g) fresh basil leaves

1 fresh small red (serrano) chilli, thinly sliced

100g buffalo mozzarella, roughly torn

1 tbsp olive oil

1 tbsp finely grated lemon rind or thin strips (see tips)

1 tbsp lemon juice

1 Preheat oven to 200°C (180°C fan/400°F/Gas 6). Line two oven trays with baking paper; mark a 22cm round on each sheet of paper, turn the paper over.

2 Process the broccoli until finely chopped. Transfer to a microwave-safe bowl, cover with plastic wrap (cling film); microwave on HIGH (100%) for 12 minutes or until tender (you can steam the broccoli instead, but do not boil it as this will make the crust too soggy). Drain. When cool enough to handle, place the broccoli in the centre of a clean tea towel; gather the ends together, then squeeze out as much excess moisture as possible.

3 Place the broccoli in a large bowl with the vegetarian cheddar, egg, and ¼ cup (20g) of the vegetarian parmesan; stir to combine. Season with salt and pepper. Divide the broccoli mixture between the two trays; spread the mixture inside the marked rounds, smooth the surface. Bake the bases for 25 minutes or until golden.

4 Spread the bases with passata, top with half the courgette and half the basil, the chilli, mozzarella, and remaining vegetarian parmesan. Bake for 20 minutes or until golden and crisp.

5 Meanwhile, combine the olive oil, lemon rind, lemon juice, remaining courgette, and remaining basil in a medium bowl; season with salt and pepper.

6 Serve the pizzas topped with the courgette salad.

TIP

If you have one, use a zester to create strips of lemon rind. If you don't, peel two long, wide strips of rind from the lemon, without the white pith, then cut them lengthways into thin strips.

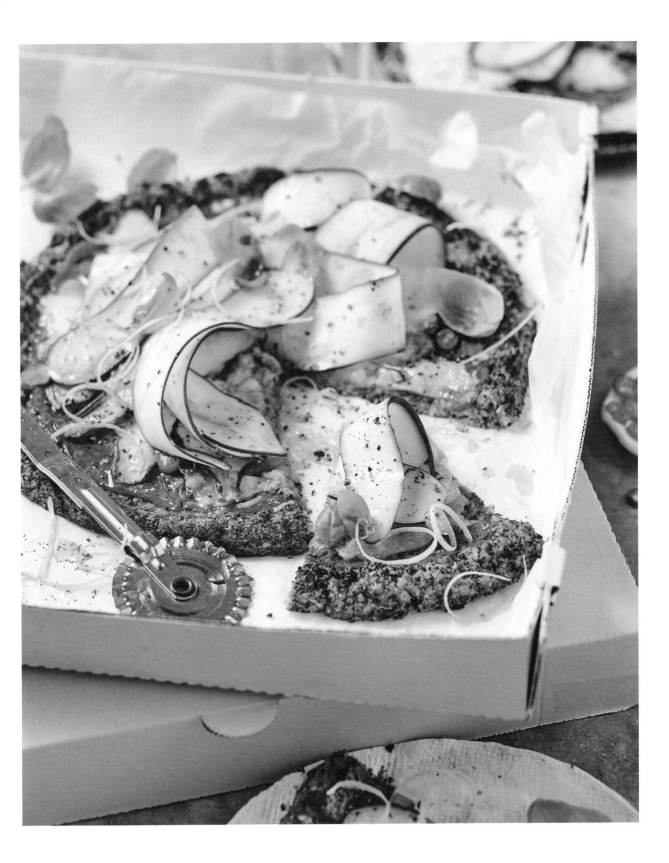

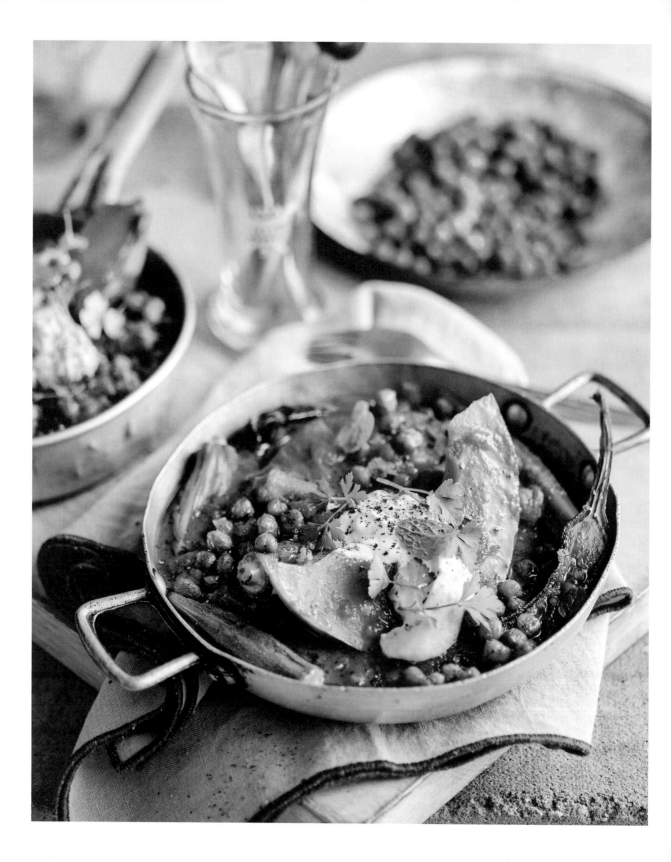

Vegetable tagine

LACTO VEGETARIAN | PREP + COOK TIME **1 HOUR + STANDING** | SERVES **4**

Tagines were traditionally cooked in the residual heat of bakers' ovens in Morocco in conical clay pots that give the dish its name. This mouthwatering veggie version is packed with warm Moroccan flavours – a perfect balance of savoury, sweet, and spicy.

2 tsp olive oil

1 large red onion (300g), coarsely chopped

2 garlic cloves, crushed

4 baby aubergines (240g), halved lengthways

500g Japanese pumpkin (kabocha squash), cut into thin wedges

2 tsp ground cumin

2 tsp ground coriander

2 tsp ground ginger

1/2 tsp ground cinnamon

400g can chopped tomatoes

2 cups (500ml) vegetable stock

2 cups (500ml) water

300g okra, trimmed

1 tbsp harissa (see tip)

3/4 cup (200g) Greek yogurt

1/2 cup (18g) finely chopped fresh flat-leaf parsley

1/2 cup (24g) finely chopped fresh mint

salt and freshly ground black pepper

harissa chickpeas

400g can chickpeas, drained, rinsed

1 tbsp harissa

1 tbsp olive oil

1 To make the harissa chickpeas, preheat oven to 200°C (180°C fan/400°F/ Gas 6). Oil a large oven tray; line with baking paper. Pat the chickpeas dry with paper towel; place in a medium bowl. Add the remaining ingredients to the chickpeas; stir to combine. Season with salt and pepper. Spread the chickpeas in a single layer on the tray. Bake for 20 minutes, stirring three times during cooking, or until well browned and slightly crunchy.

2 Heat the olive oil in a large saucepan over a medium heat; cook the onion and garlic, stirring, for 5 minutes. Add the aubergine and pumpkin; cook for 1 minute each side or until the vegetables are lightly browned. Add the spices; cook for 1 minute or until fragrant. Add the tomatoes, stock, and water; bring to the boil. Reduce heat; simmer, covered, for 15 minutes or until the vegetables are just tender.

3 Meanwhile, boil, steam, or microwave the okra until tender; drain. Stir the okra into the tagine.

4 Fold the harissa through the yogurt in a small bowl; season with salt and pepper to taste.

5 Serve the tagine topped with the yogurt mixture, harissa chickpeas, and herbs. Season with more pepper.

TIP

Harissa is a hot chilli paste. If you have a low heat-level tolerance, try using a mild chilli sauce instead or omit from the recipe.

Veggie stocks

OVO VEGETARIAN

Stock is simple to prepare and will boost the flavour of any dish. The key to preparing flavoursome stocks is a gentle simmer. If you boil the stock you will not create a well-developed flavour.

Basic vegetable stock

PREP TIME **2 HOURS 30 MINUTES** | MAKES **10 CUPS (2.5 LITRES)**

Coarsely chop 1 medium (350g) leek, 1 large (200g) unpeeled brown onion, 2 large (360g) carrots, 1 large (400g) swede, 2 celery stalks (with leaves) (300g), and 3 unpeeled garlic cloves. Place the vegetables in a boiler with 1 teaspoon of black peppercorns, 1 bouquet garni, and 20 cups (5 litres) of water; bring to the boil. Reduce heat; simmer, uncovered, for 2 hours. Strain the stock through a sieve into a large heatproof bowl; discard solids. Allow stock to cool. Cover; refrigerate until cold.

Asian-style stock

PREP TIME **2 HOURS 30 MINUTES** | MAKES **10 CUPS (2.5 LITRES)**

Coarsely chop 1 medium (350g) leek, 2 large (360g) carrots, 2 celery stalks (with leaves) (300g), 3 unpeeled garlic cloves, 10cm piece of fresh ginger, and 4 green onions (spring onions). Place the ingredients in a boiler with 1 teaspoon of black peppercorns, 20 sprigs fresh coriander, 1 cinnamon stick, 3 whole star anise, $1/2$ cup (125ml) tamari, and 20 cups (5 litres) of water. Cook following the directions for basic vegetable stock.

Italian-style stock

PREP TIME **2 HOURS 30 MINUTES** | MAKES **10 CUPS (2.5 LITRES)**

Coarsely chop 2 large (400g) unpeeled brown onions, 2 large (360g) carrots, 2 celery stalks (with leaves) (300g), and 3 unpeeled garlic cloves. Place the ingredients in a boiler with 1 teaspoon of black peppercorns, 1 bouquet garni (see tips), 1 vegetarian parmesan rind, 1 teaspoon of fennel seeds, 400g can whole peeled tomatoes, and 20 cups (5 litres) of water. Cook following the directions for basic vegetable stock.

TIPS

- To make a bouquet garni, tie 3 fresh bay leaves, 2 sprigs fresh rosemary, 6 sprigs fresh thyme, and 6 fresh flat-leaf parsley stalks together with kitchen string.
- Prepare your stock a day ahead and leave overnight before you strain it, to allow the flavours to infuse.

CLOCKWISE from top

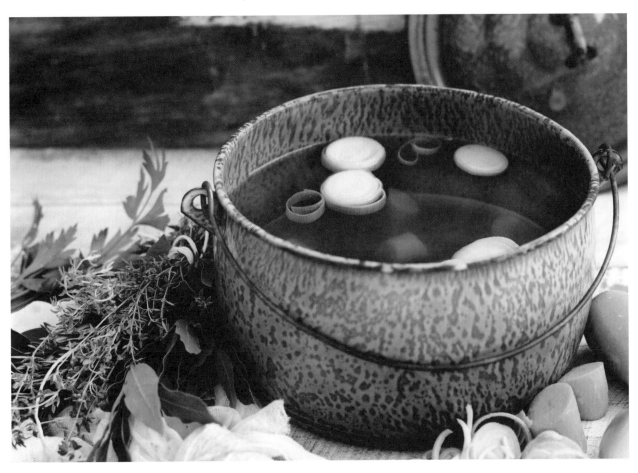

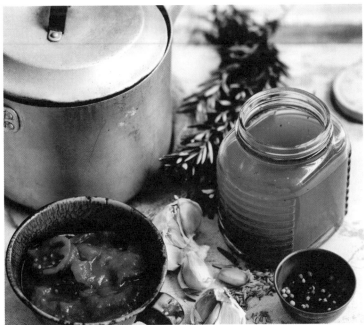

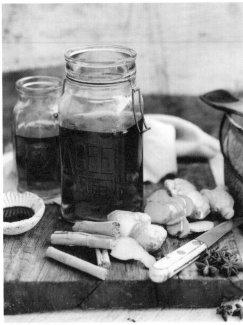

Spelt pasta with silky cauliflower sauce

LACTO VEGETARIAN | PREP + COOK TIME **40 MINUTES** | SERVES **4**

This silky cauliflower sauce can also be served with grilled seafood or chicken. Alternatively, you could reduce the amount of milk used to ¼ cup (60ml) to make a thicker cauliflower mash rather than a puree, which can be served as a side dish.

1kg cauliflower, cut into florets

1 cup (250ml) vegetable stock

2 garlic cloves, peeled

2 tbsp extra virgin olive oil

¾ cup (45g) multigrain breadcrumbs

1 fresh long red chilli, seeded, finely chopped

1 garlic clove, extra, crushed

¼ cup (6g) chopped fresh flat-leaf parsley

1 tbsp finely grated lemon rind

375g dried spelt fettuccine pasta

½ cup (40g) grated vegetarian parmesan (make sure it doesn't contain animal rennet)

2 tbsp extra virgin olive oil, extra

1½ cups (375ml) milk

¾ cup (60g) grated vegetarian parmesan, extra

1 tbsp lemon juice

salt and freshly ground black pepper

1   Place three-quarters of the cauliflower in a medium saucepan with the stock and garlic; bring to the boil. Reduce heat; simmer, covered, for 10 minutes or until the cauliflower is tender.

2   Meanwhile, cut the remaining cauliflower into tiny florets. Heat the olive oil in a large frying pan over a high heat, add the florets; cook, stirring, for 2 minutes until lightly golden. Add the breadcrumbs, chilli, and extra garlic; cook, stirring, for 2 minutes, or until the breadcrumbs are golden and crisp. Remove from the heat; stir in the parsley and lemon rind.

3   Cook the pasta in a large saucepan of boiling salted water following packet instructions. Drain well; return to the pan with the vegetarian parmesan and extra olive oil.

4   Blend the cauliflower stock mixture with the milk until very smooth. Stir in the extra vegetarian parmesan and lemon juice. Season with salt and pepper to taste.

5   Spoon the cauliflower sauce over the pasta; serve topped with the cauliflower crumbs.

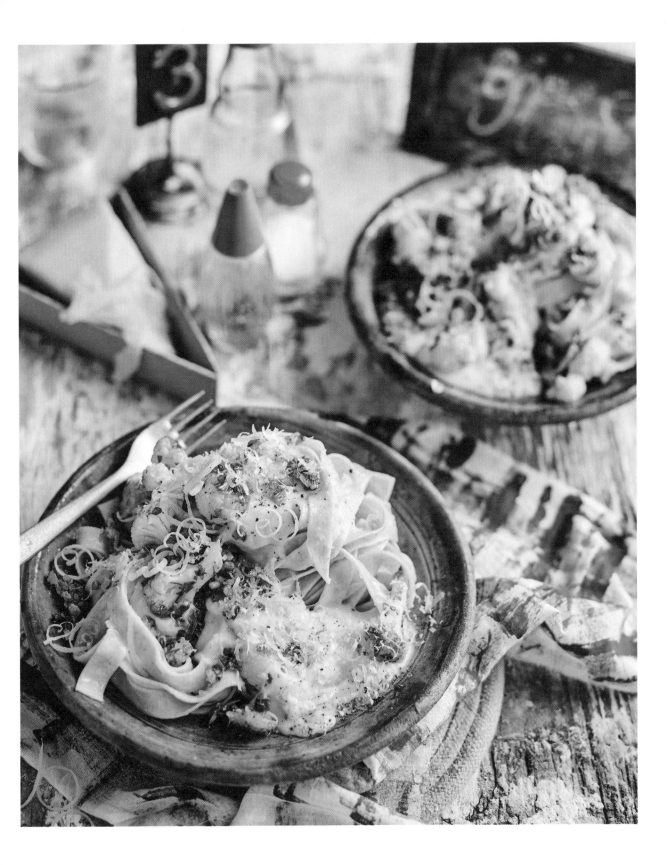

Potato and egg rendang

OVO VEGETARIAN | PREP + COOK TIME **30 MINUTES** | SERVES **4**

Rendang is a richly flavoured coconut curry popular across Southeast Asia. Typically, beef is cooked in spices then simmered in coconut milk. This veggie version retains all the deep aromatic flavours and can be cooked in a fraction of the time. Serve with steamed rice or roti.

8 small potatoes (750g), coarsely chopped

2 tbsp vegetable oil

1 medium brown onion (150g), finely chopped

185g rendang curry paste

270ml coconut milk

1/3 cup (80ml) water

salt and freshly ground black pepper

1 tbsp vegetable oil, extra

4 eggs

1 cup (16g) fresh coriander leaves

1 Boil, steam, or microwave the potatoes until just tender; drain.

2 Meanwhile, heat the oil in a medium saucepan over a medium heat; cook the onion and curry paste, stirring, for 3 minutes or until the onion has softened and the paste is fragrant.

3 Stir in the coconut milk and water; bring to a simmer. Add the potato; cook for 5 minutes, stirring occasionally. Press the potatoes lightly to crush slightly. Season with salt and pepper to taste.

4 Heat the extra oil in a large frying pan over a medium-high heat. Break the eggs into the pan; cook the eggs until done as desired.

5 Divide the curry between serving bowls; top with the fried eggs and coriander.

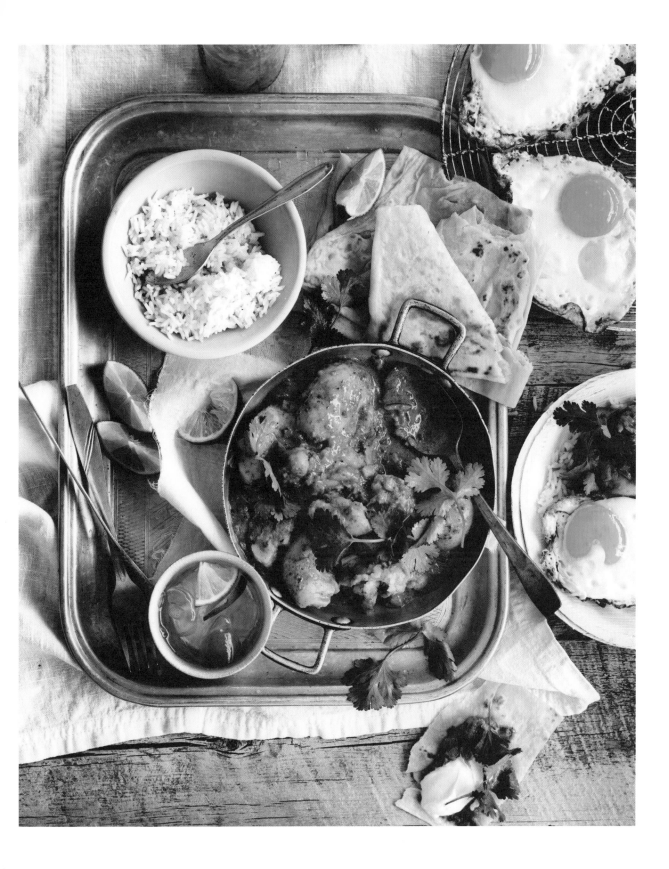

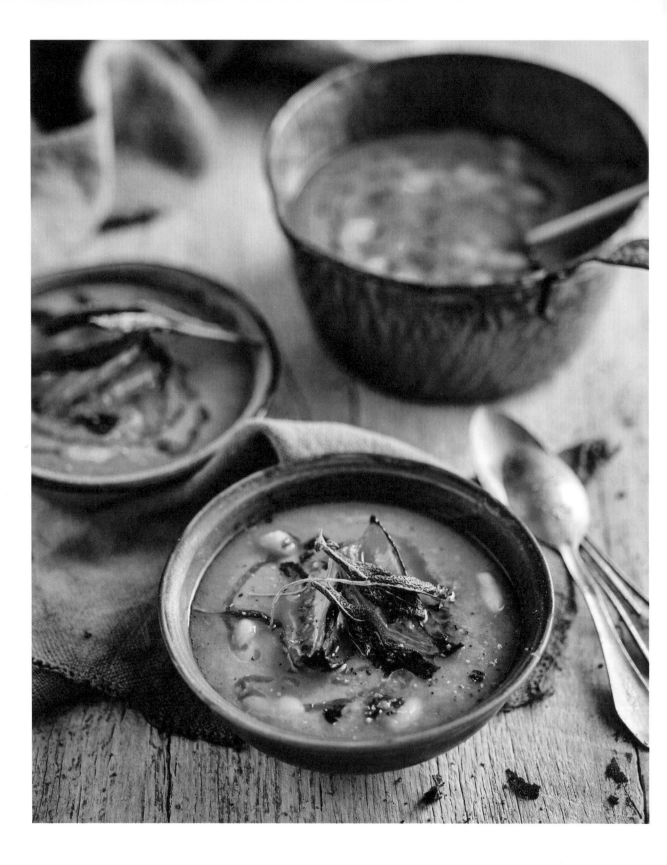

Roasted tomato and white bean soup

VEGAN | PREP + COOK TIME **1 HOUR 10 MINUTES** | SERVES **4**

Tomatoes contain the carotenoid lycopene, an antioxidant that gives them their red colour, and may be useful in reducing the risk of some cancers and heart disease. While cooking does slightly reduce the vitamin C content in tomatoes, it actually increases the lycopene content.

1kg ripe roma (plum) tomatoes, quartered

1 medium red onion (170g), cut into wedges

6 garlic cloves, unpeeled

1 tbsp pure maple syrup

1/2 cup (125ml) extra virgin olive oil

salt and freshly ground black pepper

1/3 cup (6g) loosely packed sage leaves

400g can cannellini beans, drained, rinsed

2 cups (500ml) water

1   Preheat oven to 200°C (180°C fan/400°F/Gas 6).

2   Place the tomatoes, onion, and garlic in a roasting pan. Combine the maple syrup and half the olive oil in a bowl, season with salt and pepper to taste; pour over the vegetables, then toss to coat. Roast for 45 minutes or until the tomatoes are very soft and coloured at the edges.

3   Meanwhile, heat the remaining olive oil in a small frying pan over a medium heat; fry the sage leaves, stirring, for 1 minute or until crisp. Remove with a slotted spoon; drain on paper towel. Reserve the sage oil.

4   Peel the roasted garlic. Blend the garlic, onion, two-thirds of the tomatoes, and two-thirds of the beans until smooth. Pour the mixture into a large saucepan with the water and the remaining beans; cook over a medium heat, stirring occasionally, until warmed through. Season with salt and pepper to taste.

5   Ladle the soup into bowls. Top with the remaining tomatoes and crisp sage leaves; drizzle with the reserved sage oil.

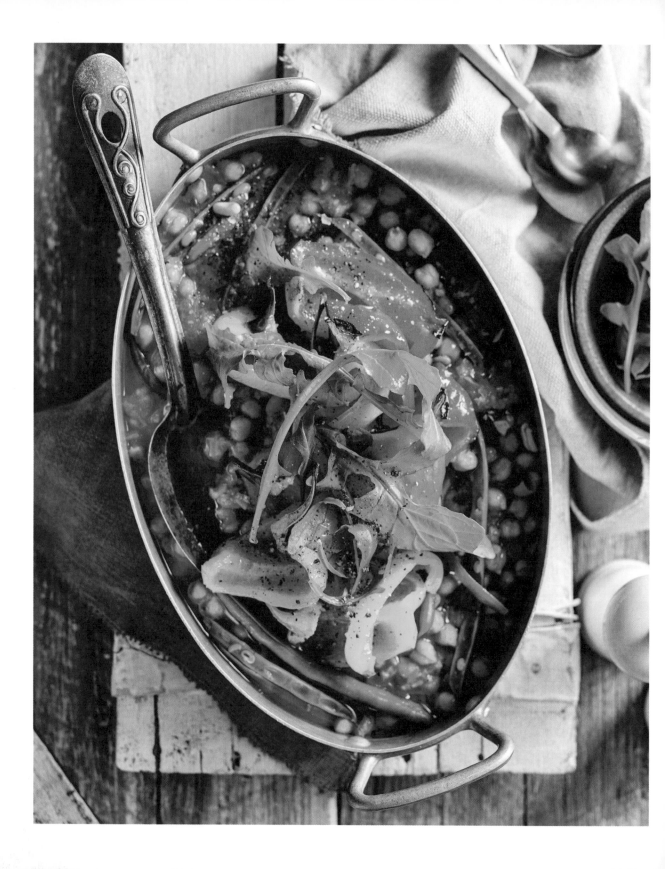

Smoky chickpea stew

VEGAN | PREP + COOK TIME **40 MINUTES** | SERVES **4**

Chickpeas are high in protein so are a fantastic alternative to meat. Highly versatile, they can be added to soups, stir-fries, and salads, and bring a nutty robustness to stews. Serve with grilled flatbread or couscous and Greek yogurt.

1 small red capsicum (pepper) (150g), quartered lengthways

1 small yellow capsicum (pepper) (150g), quartered lengthways

¼ cup (60ml) extra virgin olive oil

1 medium red onion, finely chopped

2 garlic cloves, finely chopped

3 tsp smoked paprika

pinch of saffron threads

1 cinnamon stick

2 x 400g can chickpeas, drained, rinsed

400g can chopped tomatoes

2 cups (500ml) vegetable stock

200g green beans, halved lengthways

salt and freshly ground black pepper

100g baby rocket leaves

1 Preheat oven to 220°C (200°C fan/425°F/Gas 7).

2 Place the capsicum pieces on an oven tray; drizzle with 2 tablespoons of olive oil. Roast for 15 minutes or until tender.

3 Meanwhile, heat another tablespoon of the oil in a deep, large frying pan over a medium heat; cook the onion and garlic, stirring, for 5 minutes or until soft. Add the paprika, saffron, and cinnamon; cook, stirring, for 1 minute or until fragrant.

4 Add the chickpeas, tomatoes, and stock to the pan; bring to the boil. Reduce heat; simmer over a low heat for 12 minutes or until sauce thickens. Add beans; simmer, for 2 minutes or until just tender. Season with salt and pepper to taste.

5 Serve the stew topped with capsicum and rocket, drizzled with the remaining olive oil. Finish with a good grinding of pepper.

Paneer, chickpea, and vegetable curry

LACTO VEGETARIAN | PREP + COOK TIME **30 MINUTES** | SERVES **4**

Paneer is a fresh unripened cow's milk cheese, originating in India, that is similar to pressed ricotta. It has no added salt and doesn't melt at normal cooking temperatures. You could use tofu as a substitute, if you like.

peanut oil, for shallow-frying

6 curry leaf sprigs (6g)

2 tbsp peanut oil, extra

1 large brown onion (200g), thinly sliced

2 garlic cloves, thinly sliced

1 tbsp finely grated fresh ginger

$1/3$ cup (100g) balti curry paste

400g can chickpeas, drained, rinsed

400g can chopped tomatoes

$1/2$ cup (125ml) water

400g paneer (see tip)

150g green beans, halved crossways on the diagonal

$1/4$ cup (60ml) single cream

1 Heat the peanut oil in a medium saucepan over a high heat; shallow-fry 4 curry leaf sprigs for 10 seconds or until crisp. Drain on paper towel.

2 Heat half of the extra oil in a large saucepan over a high heat; cook the onion, garlic, and ginger, stirring, for 3 minutes or until the onion softens. Add the curry paste and remaining curry leaves; cook, stirring, for 1 minute or until fragrant.

3 Add the chickpeas, tomatoes, and water; bring to the boil. Reduce heat to low; simmer, covered, for 5 minutes.

4 Meanwhile, cut the paneer into 3cm pieces. Heat the remaining oil in a large frying pan over a medium heat; cook the paneer, turning, until browned all over. Remove from pan; cool. Roughly crumble the paneer.

5 Add the beans and cream to the curry; cook for 5 minutes or until the beans are tender. Stir in the paneer; cook until heated through. Serve topped with the fried curry leaves.

TIP

Paneer is available in many major supermarkets (near the feta and haloumi) and from Indian food stores.

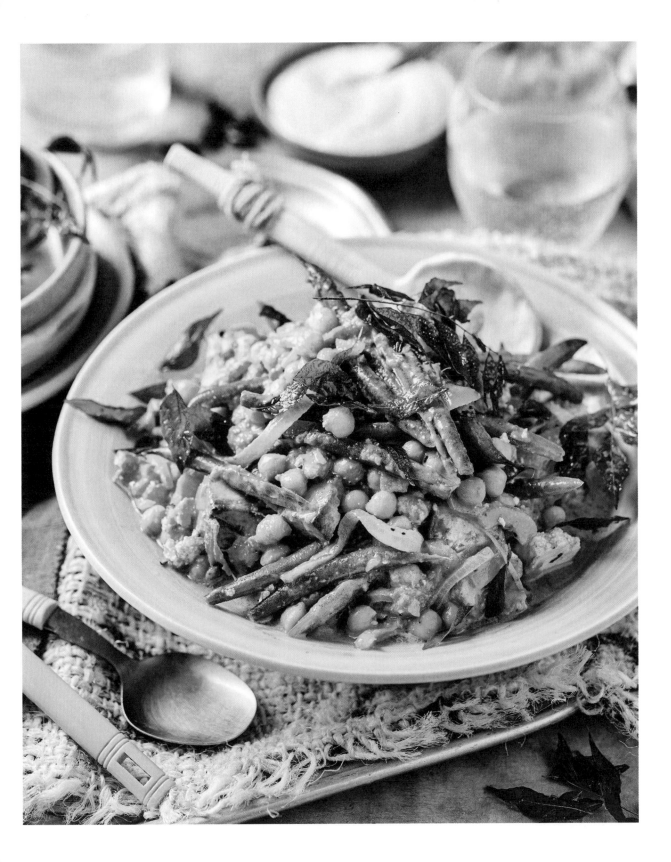

Spinach and ricotta pasta bake

LACTO VEGETARIAN | PREP + COOK TIME **1 HOUR + COOLING** | SERVES **4**

Creamy ricotta and spinach are combined in pasta shells, topped with cheese, and baked until bubbly and golden. You can make this recipe 3 hours ahead – simply cover the dishes with foil and refrigerate until you're ready to bake. Serve with a radicchio salad.

32 large pasta shells (280g)

500g spinach, stems removed

600g ricotta

2 tbsp finely chopped fresh flat-leaf parsley

1 tbsp finely chopped fresh mint

$2^2/_3$ cups (700g) bottled tomato pasta sauce

$^1/_2$ cup (125ml) vegetable stock

2 tbsp finely grated vegetarian parmesan

$^1/_4$ cup (3g) small fresh basil leaves

1 Cook the pasta shells in a large saucepan of boiling water for 3 minutes; drain. Cool for 10 minutes. Transfer to a tray.

2 Preheat oven to 180°C (160°C fan/350°F/Gas 4). Oil four 2-cup (500ml) shallow ovenproof dishes.

3 Boil, steam, or microwave the spinach until wilted; drain. Rinse under cold running water; drain. Squeeze the excess liquid from the spinach; chop finely.

4 Place the spinach in a large bowl with the ricotta and herbs; stir to combine. Spoon the mixture into the pasta shells.

5 Combine the tomato sauce and stock in a jug; pour into the dishes. Place the filled pasta shells in the dishes; sprinkle with half the vegetarian parmesan. Cover the dishes with foil; place on an oven tray.

6 Bake for 30 minutes or until the pasta is tender. Remove foil; bake for a further 10 minutes. Cool for 10 minutes. Serve the pasta bake topped with the remaining vegetarian parmesan and basil.

TIP

This recipe can be made in a shallow 2-litre (8-cup) ovenproof dish. Bake, covered with foil, for 50 minutes or until the pasta is tender; remove the foil, then bake for a further 10 minutes.

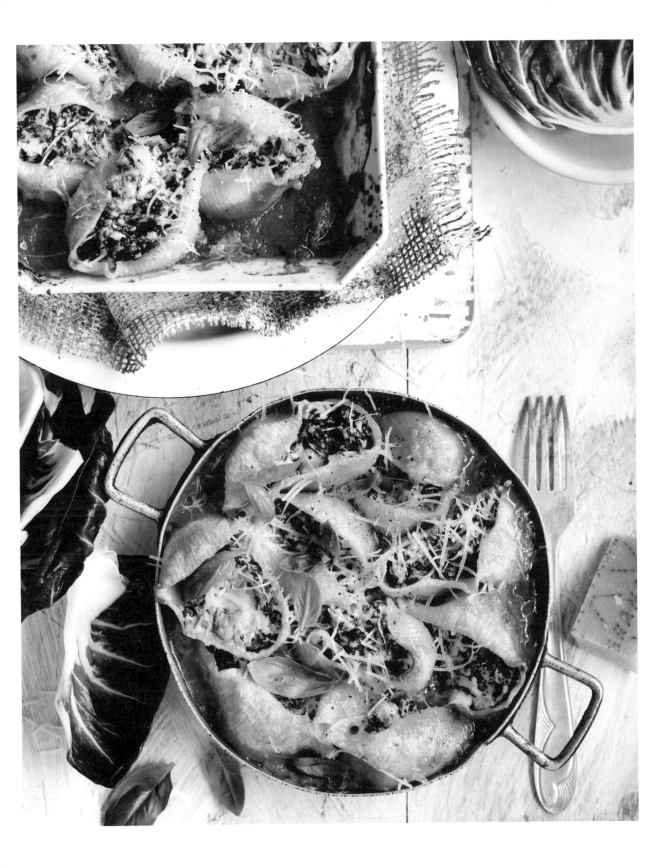

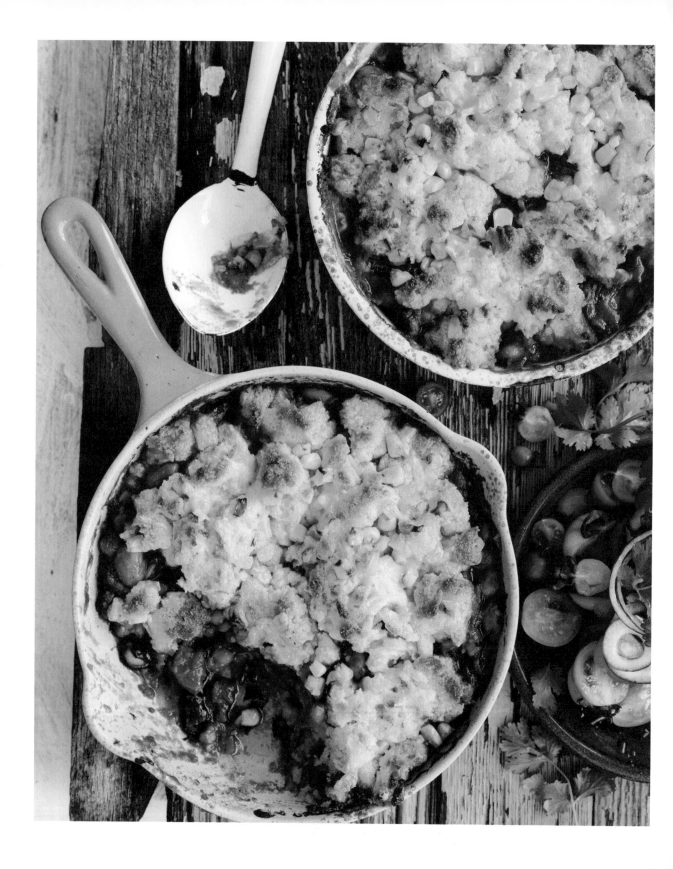

Chilli bean pie with cornbread crust

LACTO-OVO VEGETARIAN | PREP + COOK TIME **1 HOUR** | SERVES **6**

This flavourful 4-bean chilli is taken to the next level by its golden cheesy cornbread and sweetcorn topping. The hearty nutritious beans and chilli kick make this the perfect comforting winter warmer.

2 tbsp olive oil

1 medium brown onion (150g), finely chopped

1 medium green capsicum (pepper) (200g), finely chopped

2 garlic cloves, crushed

2 tsp Mexican chilli powder

1 tsp ground cumin

2 x 400g cans chopped tomatoes

1½ cups (375ml) vegetable stock

4 x 400g cans four bean mix, drained, rinsed

¼ cup (8g) finely chopped fresh coriander

salt and freshly ground black pepper

¾ cup (110g) self-raising flour

¾ cup (125g) polenta

90g butter, coarsely chopped

1 egg, lightly beaten

⅓ cup (40g) coarsely grated vegetarian cheddar

125g canned corn kernels (sweetcorn), drained

2 tbsp milk, approximately

tomato and lime salsa

400g mixed baby heirloom tomatoes, halved

½ cup (8g) fresh coriander leaves

½ small red onion (50g), finely sliced

2 tbsp lime juice

1 Heat the oil in a large saucepan over a medium-high heat; cook the onion, capsicum, and garlic, stirring, for 5 minutes or until the onion softens. Add the chilli and cumin; cook, stirring, for 1 minute or until fragrant. Add the tomatoes, stock, and bean mix; bring to the boil. Reduce heat; simmer, uncovered, for 15 minutes or until the sauce has thickened slightly. Stir in the coriander; season with salt and pepper to taste.

2 Meanwhile, preheat oven to 200°C (180°C fan/400°F/Gas 6). Place the flour and polenta in a medium bowl; rub in the butter. Stir in the egg, cheddar, half the corn, and enough milk to make a soft, sticky dough.

3 Spoon the bean mixture into a 2-litre (8-cup) ovenproof dish. Drop tablespoons of the corn mixture on top of the bean mixture; top with the remaining corn. Bake for 20 minutes or until browned.

4 Meanwhile, to make the tomato and lime salsa, combine the ingredients in a small bowl. Season with salt and pepper to taste.

5 Serve the chilli bean pie with the salsa.

Green shakshuka

LACTO-OVO VEGETARIAN | PREP + COOK TIME **30 MINUTES** | SERVES **4**

Traditional shakshuka originates from North Africa. It's a simple one-pot dish of gently poached eggs in a tasty mixture of simmering vegetables. You can use silverbeet (Swiss chard) or spinach instead of the kale, if you prefer. Serve with a radicchio salad.

2 tbsp olive oil

1 medium leek (350g), thinly sliced

1 garlic clove, thinly sliced

1 baby fennel bulb (130g), trimmed, thinly sliced, fronds reserved

150g green kale, coarsely chopped

½ cup (125ml) vegetable stock

8 eggs

salt and freshly ground black pepper

½ cup (125g) labneh

¼ cup (60g) halved spicy green olives

¼ tsp ground sumac

4 pita pocket breads (150g)

1 Heat the olive oil in a large frying pan over a medium heat; cook the leek, garlic, fennel, and kale, stirring occasionally, for 5 minutes or until the vegetables soften. Stir in the stock; bring to a simmer.

2 Using the back of a spoon, make eight shallow indents in the mixture. Break 1 egg into each hole. Cook, covered, over a low heat, for 6 minutes or until the egg whites are set and yolks remain runny, or until cooked to your liking. Season with salt and pepper.

3 Top the shakshuka with labneh and olives; sprinkle with the sumac and reserved fennel fronds. Serve with char-grilled pita bread.

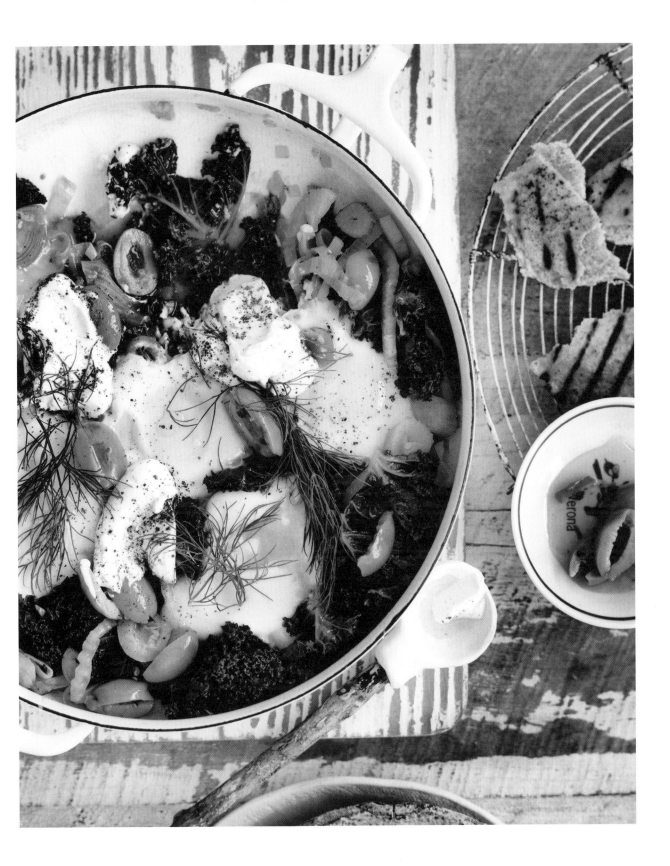

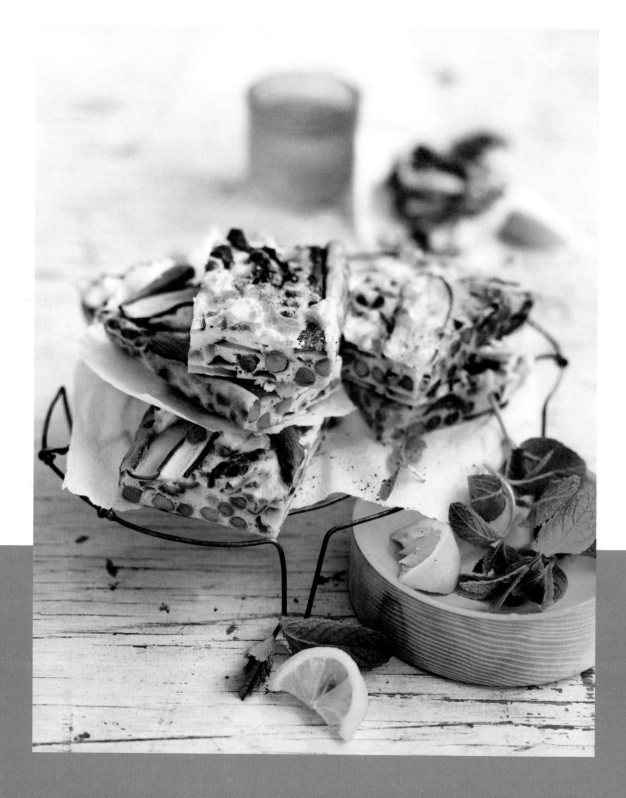

FOOD
TO SHARE

Too good to be enjoyed alone, these fresh,
balanced dishes are perfect for entertaining.
Serve as a sharing platter for lunch with
friends or as finger food at a party.

Spiced paneer and aubergine fritters

LACTO VEGETARIAN | PREP + COOK TIME **1 HOUR** | SERVES **6**

Spicy, fragrant, crispy on the outside and mouthwateringly soft and melting on the inside, these golden fritters are packed with Indian flavours and make for a delicious platter of nibbles to pass around a party. Serve with any chutney of your choice.

1 large aubergine (500g), cut into 2.5cm pieces

2 tbsp vegetable oil

1 tbsp cumin seeds

salt and freshly ground black pepper

2 cups (300g) chickpea flour

1 tbsp ground coriander

2 tsp garam masala

1½ cups (375ml) water

200g paneer, cut into 2.5cm pieces

vegetable oil, extra, for deep-frying

1 medium lime (65g), cut in half or wedges

coconut mint chutney

1 cup (8g) fresh mint leaves, extra

1 cup (16g) fresh coriander leaves

½ cup (125ml) water

½ cup (40g) shredded coconut

2 green onions (spring onions), coarsely chopped

1 fresh long green chilli, coarsely chopped

2 tbsp lime juice

1 tsp ground cumin

1 Preheat oven to 200°C (180°C fan/400°F/Gas 6). Line a roasting pan with baking paper. Combine the aubergine, vegetable oil, and cumin seeds in a pan; season with salt and pepper. Roast for 30 minutes, stirring halfway through cooking time, or until golden. Reduce oven to 100°C (80°C /210°F).

2 Meanwhile, to make the coconut mint chutney, process the ingredients until smooth. Season with salt and pepper to taste.

3 Whisk the chickpea flour, ground coriander, and garam masala in a medium bowl to combine. Whisk in the water until just combined. Season with salt and pepper. Stir in the aubergine and paneer.

4 Fill a large saucepan one-third full with extra oil; heat to 180°C (160°C fan/350°F/Gas 4) (or until a cube of bread browns in 10 seconds). Deep-fry individual pieces of aubergine and paneer, in three batches, allowing excess batter to drain off before adding to the oil, for 3 minutes, turning halfway through cooking, or until golden. Remove with a slotted spoon; drain on paper towel. Season with salt.

5 Serve the fritters with the chutney and lime wedges.

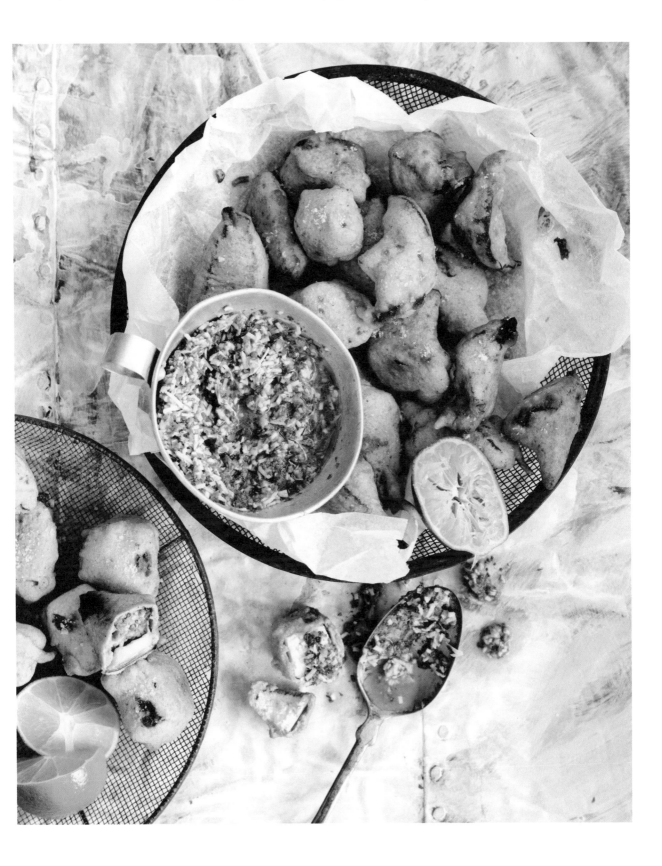

Baked brie with pine nut dukkah

LACTO VEGETARIAN | PREP + COOK TIME **20 MINUTES** | SERVES **6**

Dukah is an Egyptian nut, seed, and spice blend that can enliven many an appetizer or sharing platter. Any leftover dukkah can be sprinkled on salads, soft cheese, or roasted vegetables, or simply serve with bread and oil.

280g whole double brie cheese

1 garlic clove, thinly sliced

1 tbsp pomegranate molasses (see tip)

50g dried muscatel raisins (see tip)

100g lavosh crackers (see tip)

pine nut dukkah

$1/4$ cup (40g) pine nuts

$1/4$ cup (40g) blanched almonds

1 tbsp sesame seeds

1 tsp cumin seeds

1 tsp coriander seeds

salt and freshly ground black pepper

1 Preheat oven to 180°C (160°C fan/350°F/Gas 4). Line an oven tray with baking paper.

2 Place the brie on the tray; using a small knife, cut small holes in the top of the cheese. Press the garlic slices into the holes. Bake for 15 minutes or until warm and soft.

3 Meanwhile, to make the pine nut dukkah, stir the ingredients in a small dry frying pan over a medium heat for 3 minutes, or until the nuts are golden. Process until coarsely chopped. Season with salt and pepper.

4 Drizzle the molasses over the warm brie; sprinkle with dukkah. Serve the baked brie with the muscatels and crackers.

TIP

Pomegranate molasses, muscatels, and lavosh crackers are available at Middle Eastern food stores, specialty food shops, and some delicatessens.

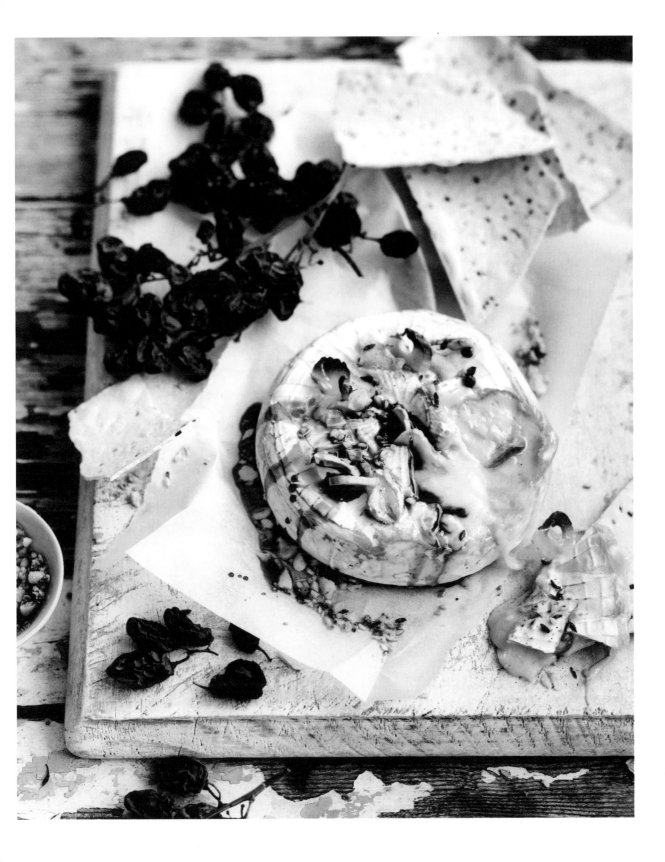

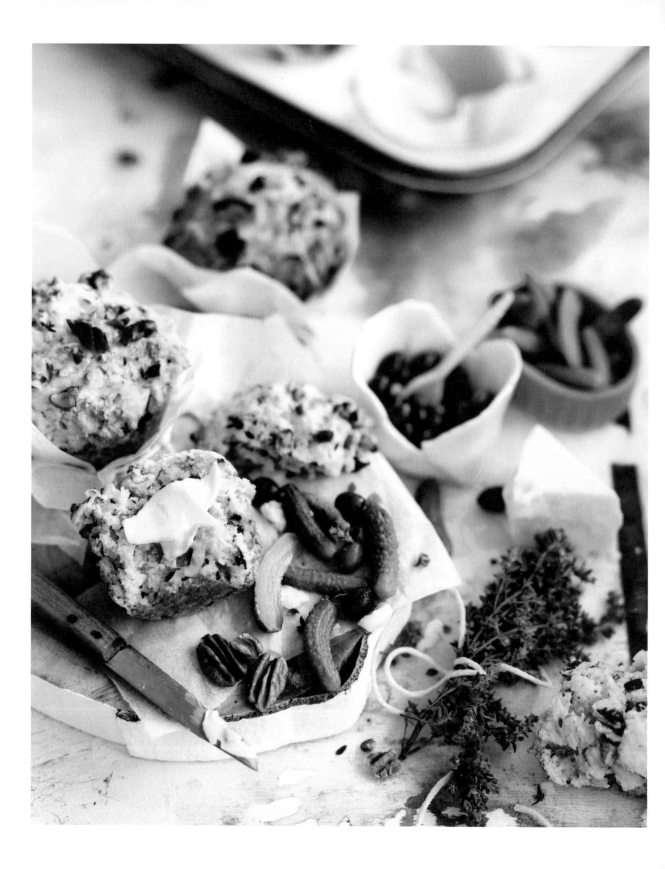

Vegetarian cheddar, thyme, and pecan muffins

LACTO-OVO VEGETARIAN | PREP + COOK TIME **45 MINUTES** | MAKES **6**

These cheesy, herby clouds of deliciousness are perfect for a sharing lunch with friends.
This mixture could also be baked in a 12-hole ($^1/_3$-cup/80ml) muffin pan. They will take about
15 minutes to cook. Spread muffins with butter, if you like.

3 cups (450g) self-raising flour

1 tsp sea salt flakes

1 tbsp finely chopped fresh thyme

2 tbsp finely chopped fresh flat-leaf parsley

100g pitted black and green olives, coarsely chopped

1$^1/_3$ cups (160g) grated vegetarian cheddar

1 cup (120g) coarsely chopped pecans

2 eggs, lightly beaten

1$^1/_4$ cups (310ml) buttermilk

$^1/_3$ cup (80ml) vegetable oil

12 sprigs fresh thyme, extra

$^1/_4$ cup (45g) drained cornichons

$^1/_3$ cup (55g) black olives, extra

100g vegetarian cheddar, extra

1   Preheat oven to 180°C (160°C fan/350°F/Gas 4). Grease and flour a 6-hole ($^3/_4$-cup/180ml) muffin pan.

2   Place the flour, salt, chopped thyme and parsley, olives, 1 cup (40g) of the vegetarian cheddar, and $^3/_4$ cup (90g) of the pecans in a large bowl; mix well. Make a well in the centre, add the combined egg, buttermilk, and vegetable oil; mix until just combined. Spoon the mixture into the pan holes; sprinkle with the remaining vegetarian cheddar, remaining pecans, and the extra thyme.

3   Bake the muffins for 25 minutes or until a skewer inserted into the centre comes out clean. Leave in the pan for 5 minutes before turning onto a wire rack.

4   Serve the muffins warm or cooled with cornichons, the extra olives, and the extra cheese.

TIP

These muffins can be frozen for up to three months.
Thaw, then warm in the oven or microwave before
serving, to refresh.

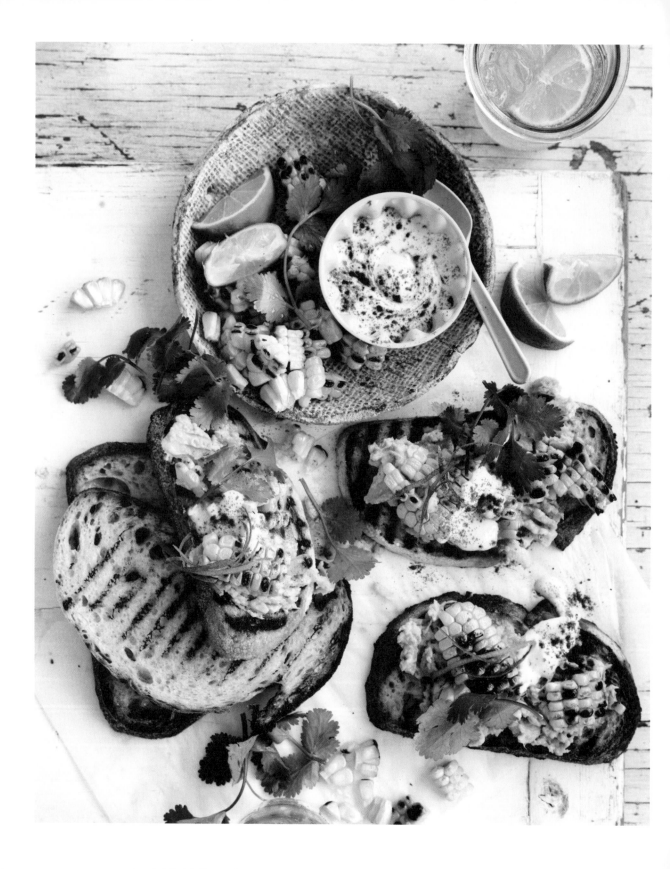

Mexican corn and avocado bruschetta

LACTO VEGETARIAN | PREP + COOK TIME **30 MINUTES** | SERVES **4**

The Italian antipasto classic is given a Mexican twist here – perfect for your party menu. The spiced lime yogurt can be made several hours ahead; store covered in the refrigerator. You could also serve topped with crumbled feta.

3 trimmed corn cobs (750g)

8 thin slices sourdough bread (450g)

¼ cup (60ml) olive oil

2 large avocados (640g), chopped

¼ cup (4g) fresh coriander leaves

1 tsp lime rind strips (see tip)

lime wedges, to serve

salt and freshly ground black pepper

spiced lime yogurt

½ cup (140g) Greek yogurt

1 garlic clove, crushed

1 tbsp lime juice

Pinch of cayenne pepper

1   Cook the corn cobs on a heated oiled grill plate (or barbecue), turning occasionally, for 15 minutes or until charred and tender. When cool enough to handle, cut the kernels from the cobs.

2   Meanwhile, to make the spiced lime yogurt, gently swirl the ingredients together in a small bowl; season with salt and pepper to taste.

3   Brush the bread with 2 tablespoons of the olive oil; place on a heated oiled grill plate (or grill or barbecue) for 1 minute each side or until lightly charred.

4   Mash the avocado in a small bowl with the remaining olive oil. Season with salt and pepper.

5   Spread the avocado on the toasted bread; season with salt and pepper. Top with the corn and the spiced lime yogurt, then the coriander and lime rind. Serve with lime wedges.

TIP

To create the thin strips of lime rind, use a zester if you have one. If you don't, peel two long, wide pieces of rind from the lime, without the white pith, then cut them lengthways into thin strips.

Pea, chickpea, and hazelnut falafel

LACTO-OVO VEGETARIAN | PREP + COOK TIME **30 MINUTES + REFRIGERATION** | MAKES **12**

Falafel is a popular street food, originating in the Middle East. Traditionally made with ground chickpeas or fava beans, this vegetarian favourite is often served with pitta or flatbread. This nutritious nutty variation works well as finger food, served with a yoghurt dip.

$^1/_2$ cup (60g) frozen peas, thawed

125g canned chickpeas, drained, rinsed

50g feta, crumbled

2 tbsp coarsely chopped fresh mint

1 fresh long green chilli, seeded, finely chopped

1 free-range egg

$^1/_4$ cup (25g) hazelnut meal (ground hazelnuts)

salt and freshly ground black pepper

1 tbsp white sesame seeds

$^1/_4$ cup (30g) finely chopped hazelnuts

vegetable oil, for shallow-frying

1 medium lemon (140g), cut into wedges

mint yogurt

$^1/_2$ cup (140g) Greek yogurt

1 tbsp lemon juice

1 tbsp finely chopped fresh mint

1 Place the peas, chickpeas, feta, mint, chilli, egg, and hazelnut meal in a food processor; pulse until coarsely chopped and combined. Season with salt and pepper. Shape tablespoons of the mixture into balls; flatten slightly. Toss the falafel in the combined sesame seeds and chopped hazelnuts. Place falafel on a baking-paper-lined oven tray. Refrigerate for 30 minutes.

2 Meanwhile, to make the mint yogurt, combine the ingredients in a small bowl.

3 Heat the vegetable oil in a medium frying pan over a medium-high heat; shallow-fry the falafel, in batches, for 5 minutes or until golden brown. Drain on paper towel.

4 Serve the falafel with mint yogurt and lemon wedges.

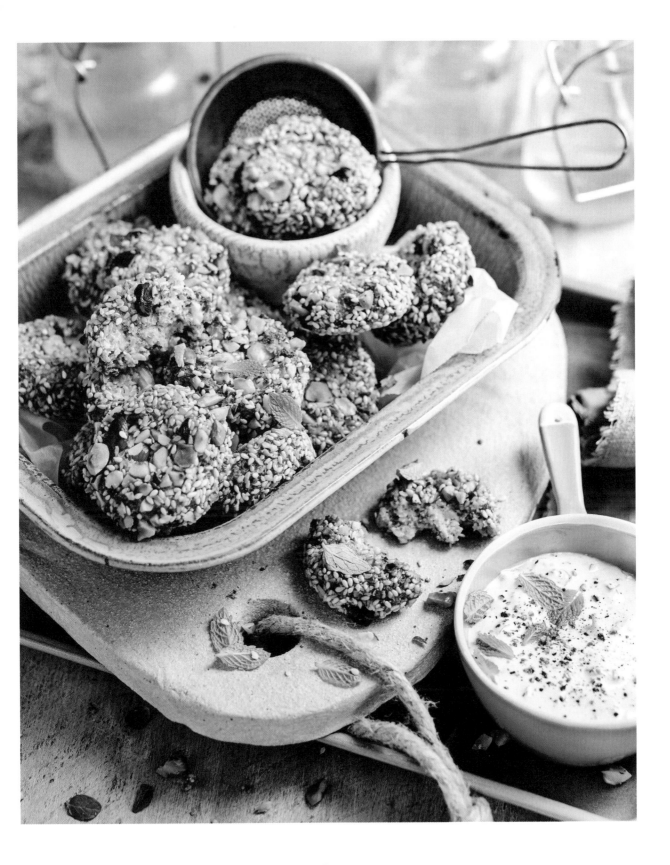

Green power mini frittatas

LACTO-OVO VEGETARIAN | PREP + COOK TIME **35 MINUTES** | MAKES **8**

These mini frittatas are packed with power greens and also pack a punch when it comes to flavour. Ideal for serving to guests the morning after the night before for a healthy, protein-rich breakfast to get everyone on track for the day ahead.

2 tsp olive oil

1 small leek (200g), thinly sliced

½ garlic clove, crushed

3 cups (120g) firmly packed baby spinach leaves, finely chopped

5 eggs

½ cup (125ml) single cream

1 tbsp finely chopped fresh mint

1 tbsp finely chopped fresh basil

1 tbsp finely chopped fresh dill

salt and freshly ground black pepper

100g feta, crumbled

1 Preheat oven to 180°C (160°C fan/350°F/Gas 4). Line 8 holes of a 12-hole (⅓ cup/80ml) muffin pan with paper cases.

2 Heat the olive oil in a medium saucepan over a medium heat; cook the leek, stirring, for 3 minutes. Add the garlic; cook for 2 minutes or until the leek is soft. Add the spinach; cook, stirring, for 30 seconds or until wilted. Remove from the heat. Set aside.

3 Whisk the eggs, cream, and herbs in a medium jug; season with salt and pepper.

4 Divide the spinach mixture into the pan holes; pour in the egg mixture, then top with feta.

5 Bake the frittatas for 20 minutes or until set. Leave in the pan for 5 minutes before serving warm or at room temperature.

TIP

Store frittatas in an airtight container in the fridge for up to 5 days or freeze for up to 1 month.

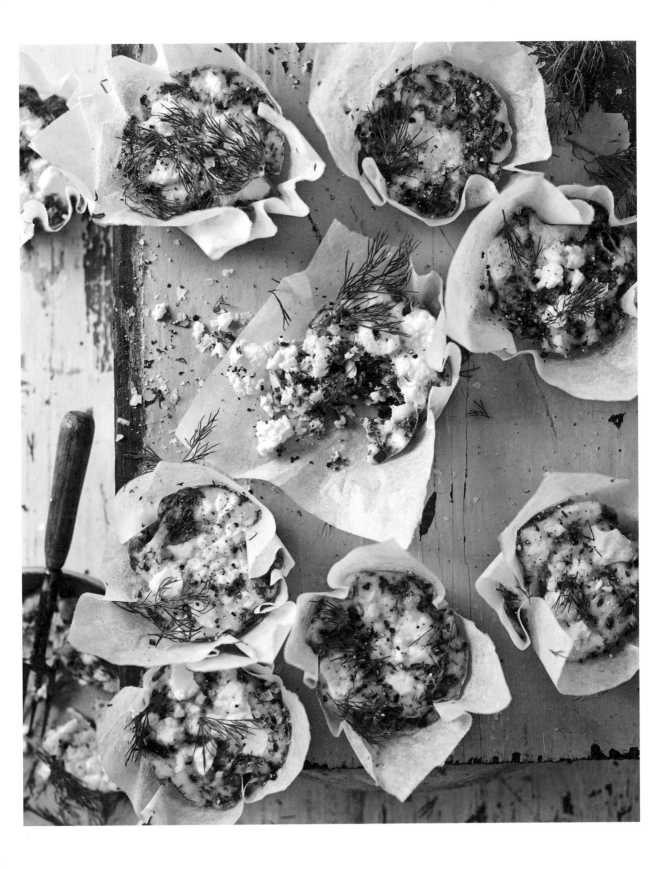

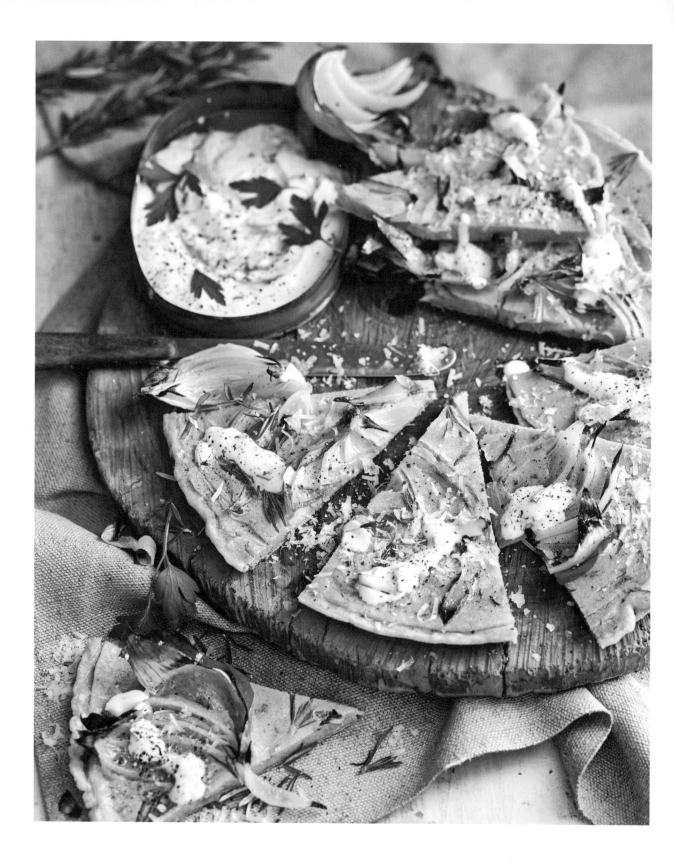

Roasted onion socca with chilli yogurt

LACTO VEGETARIAN | PREP + COOK TIME **40 MINUTES** | SERVES **8**

Socca, also known as farinata, is a traditional Italian and Provençal pancake made from
chickpea flour. It's a great source of protein and fibre and makes a wonderful light lunch.
You will need an ovenproof frying pan for this recipe.

1 medium brown onion (150g)

$1/2$ cup (125ml) olive oil

salt and freshly ground black pepper

$1^1/2$ cups (180g) chickpea flour

1 tsp salt flakes

$1^1/4$ cups (310ml) lukewarm water

2 tsp chopped fresh rosemary

1 tbsp small fresh rosemary sprigs

$1/4$ cup (20g) finely grated vegetarian parmesan
(make sure it doesn't contain animal rennet)

chilli yogurt

$1/2$ cup (140g) Greek yogurt

1 tsp raw honey

1 tbsp coarsely chopped fresh flat-leaf parsley

$1/4$ tsp chilli flake

1   Preheat oven to 200°C (180°C fan/400°F/Gas 6). Line an oven tray with baking paper.

2   Cut the onion into eight wedges; separate the layers. Place the onion in a medium bowl with 1 tablespoon of the olive oil; toss to coat. Season with salt and pepper. Place the onion on the oven tray; bake for 20 minutes or until browned.

3   Place the chickpea flour, salt, water, chopped rosemary, and $1/4$ cup (60ml) of the olive oil in a medium bowl; whisk until smooth. Season with cracked black pepper. Set aside for 5 minutes.

4   To make the chilli yogurt, combine the ingredients in a small bowl.

5   Increase oven to 250°C (230°C fan/480°F/Gas 9). Heat a large heavy-based ovenproof frying pan over a medium-high heat. Add the remaining olive oil, heat for a few seconds, pour in the batter, top with the onion and rosemary sprigs. Cook for 1 minute; transfer to the oven, bake for 10 minutes or until golden and the socca pulls away from the side of the pan.

6   Serve the socca cut into wedges, topped with the vegetarian parmesan and the chilli yogurt.

TIP

Store socca in an airtight container in the fridge
for up to 3 days or freeze for up to 1 month

Mayos

VEGAN

Finding a good-quality vegan mayonnaise is difficult and most are soy based.
This recipe is not only dairy-free and egg-free, but soy-free as well and results in
a deliciously rich, thick, creamy mayo.

Basic vegan mayo

PREP TIME **10 MINUTES + STANDING** | MAKES **2 CUPS (600g)**

Soak 1 cup (160g) whole blanched almonds for 4 hours; drain. Rinse under cold water; drain. Blend the almonds with ½ cup (125ml) of water until smooth. Add 1 tablespoon of apple cider vinegar, 1 tablespoon of lemon juice, and 1 teaspoon of dijon mustard; blend until smooth and combined. Season with salt and pepper to taste. With the motor operating, add ½ cup (125ml) olive oil in a slow, steady stream until smooth and combined. Store in an airtight container in the fridge for up to 1 month.

Aioli

PREP TIME **10 MINUTES + STANDING** | MAKES **2 CUPS (600g)**

Make basic vegan mayo on left; stir in 1 clove crushed garlic.

Harissa mayo

PREP TIME **10 MINUTES + STANDING** | MAKES **2 CUPS (600g)**

Make basic vegan mayo on left; stir in harissa to taste.

TIPS

- If the vegan mayonnaise is not tart enough for your taste, add a little more lemon juice. If it is too tart, add a little cold water.
- Spread these vegan mayonnaises on sandwiches, serve as an accompaniment with vegan recipes, as an ingredient in place of egg-based mayonnaise, or as a dip with vegetable sticks.

CLOCKWISE from top

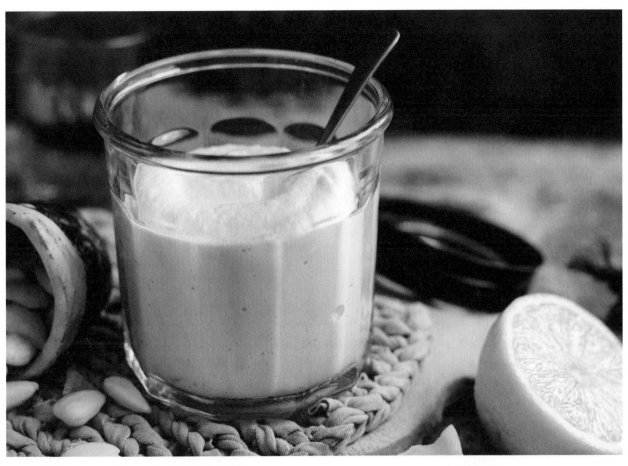

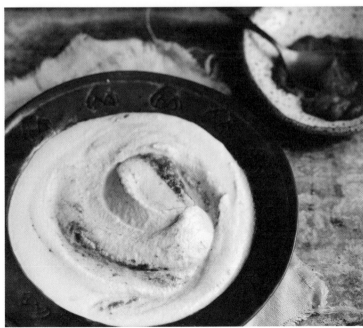

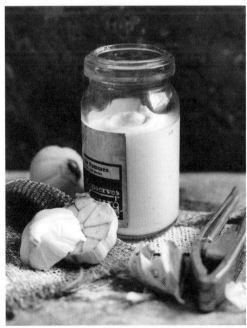

Courgette and sweet potato loaf

LACTO-OVO VEGETARIAN | PREP + COOK TIME **1 HOUR 20 MINUTES + COOLING** | SERVES **6**

Courgette adds a great texture and moistness to baked goods, as well as bringing nutritional value. Use butternut pumpkin (butternut squash) or carrot instead of the sweet potato, if you like. Serve spread with butter or herb-flavoured soft cheese or goat's cheese.

1 tbsp olive oil

1 medium brown onion (150g), finely chopped

2 garlic cloves, crushed

2 tsp finely chopped fresh rosemary

2 large courgettes (300g), coarsely grated

1 small white sweet potato (250g), coarsely grated

1 cup (150g) self-raising flour

1 cup (80g) finely grated vegetarian parmesan

1/2 tsp ground nutmeg

1 tsp cracked black pepper

5 eggs, lightly beaten

1/2 cup (125ml) buttermilk (see tip)

1/4 cup (35g) drained sun-dried tomatoes in oil, thinly sliced

1 long sprig fresh rosemary

1 Preheat oven to 180°C (160°C fan/350°F/Gas 4). Grease a 10cm x 20cm loaf pan (top measurement); line the bottom and long sides with baking paper, extending the paper 5cm over the edge.

2 Heat the olive oil in a medium frying pan over a medium heat; cook the onion, garlic, and chopped rosemary, stirring, for 4 minutes or until lightly golden. Transfer to a large bowl; cool slightly.

3 Squeeze excess liquid from the courgette. Add the courgette to the onion mixture with the sweet potato, flour, vegetarian parmesan, nutmeg, and pepper; mix to combine. Make a well in the centre, add the eggs, buttermilk, and tomatoes; mix until just combined. Spread the mixture into the pan; top with the rosemary sprig.

4 Bake the loaf for 1 hour or until browned and a skewer inserted into the centre comes out clean. Cover loosely with foil if overbrowning during cooking. Cool in the pan for 20 minutes before turning out. Serve sliced, warm or at room temperature.

TIP

If you don't have any buttermilk on hand, you can make your own: place 2 teaspoons of lemon juice in a jug and add enough low-fat milk to make it up to 1/2 cup (125ml).

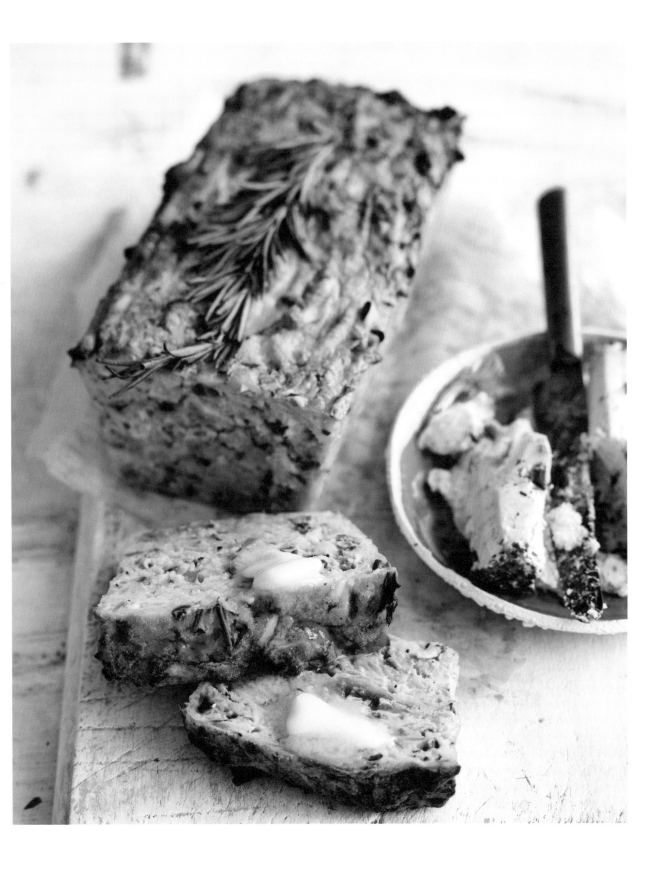

Spicy sweet potato sausage rolls

LACTO-OVO VEGETARIAN | PREP + COOK TIME **1 HOUR** | SERVES **4**

Here sausage meat is replaced with a spicy veggie filling encased in golden buttery puff pastry. You could assemble the sausage rolls ahead of time and refrigerate until ready to cook. Butternut pumpkin (butternut squash) can be used instead of sweet potato.

600g sweet potato, coarsely chopped

400g can red kidney beans, drained, rinsed

150g drained char-grilled capsicums (peppers), finely chopped

150g feta, crumbled

2 green onions (spring onions), finely chopped

½ cup (15g) finely chopped fresh coriander leaves

1 tbsp ground cumin

1 tsp dried chilli flakes

salt and freshly ground black pepper

4 sheets puff pastry, just thawed

1 free-range egg, lightly beaten

2 tsp cumin seeds

½ cup (140g) smoky barbecue sauce

1 Preheat oven to 200°C (180°C fan/400°F/Gas 6). Line two oven trays with baking paper.

2 Boil, steam, or microwave the sweet potato until tender; drain. Mash the sweet potato in a large bowl until smooth.

3 Add the beans, capsicum, and feta to the bowl with green onion, coriander, ground cumin, and chilli; mix well. Season with salt and pepper.

4 Spread a quarter of the sweet potato mixture along one side of each sheet of pastry. Roll up to enclose. Place the rolls, seam-side down, on the trays. Brush with egg; sprinkle with the cumin seeds.

5 Bake the rolls for 30 minutes or until golden and puffed. Cut each roll into four pieces; serve with barbecue sauce.

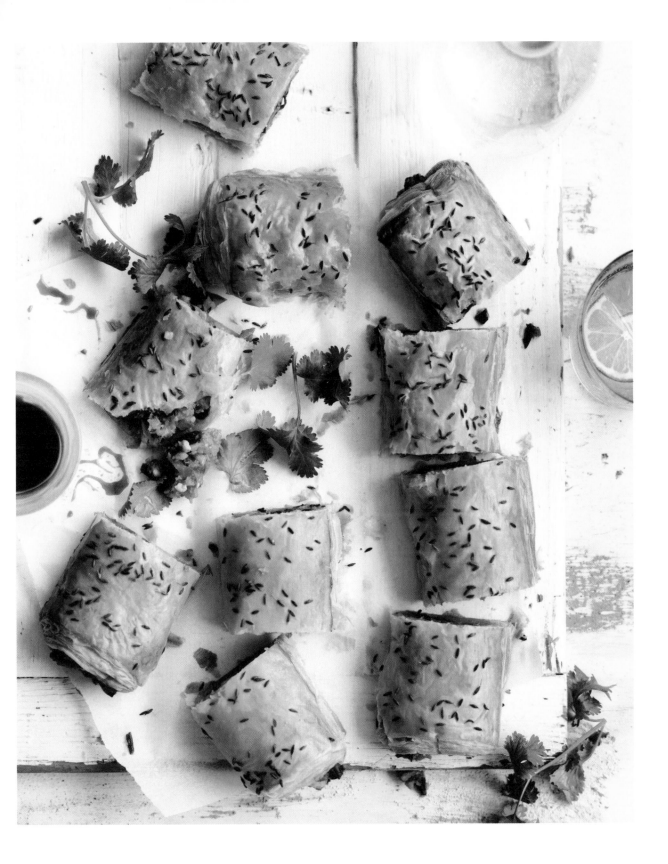

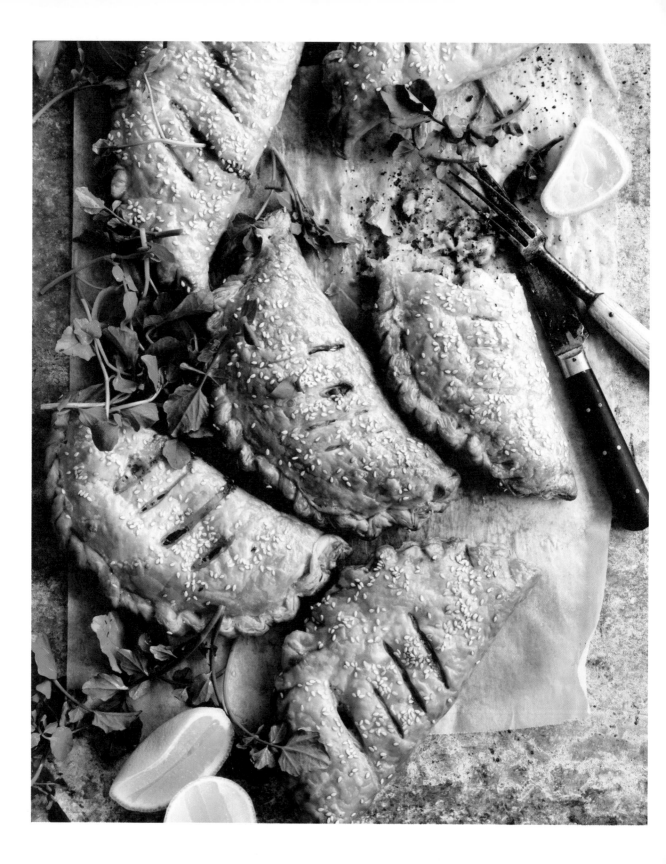

Broccoli, mustard, and cheddar hand pies

LACTO VEGETARIAN | PREP + COOK TIME **30 MINUTES** | SERVES **4**

These hand pies are bursting with cheesy flavour and have a mouthwatering mustard zing.
Ideal for a handheld lunch on the go or for a sharing platter with friends. Serve
with a simple green salad.

6 sheets puff pastry

1/2 cup (140g) honey mustard

300g broccoli, finely chopped

1 1/2 cups (180g) grated vegetarian cheddar

1 1/2 cups (150g) grated mozzarella

salt and freshly ground black pepper

1 free-range egg, lightly beaten

3 tsp toasted sesame seeds

1 Preheat oven to 200°C (180°C fan/400°F/Gas 6). Line two oven trays with baking paper.

2 Using a plate as a guide, cut six 22cm rounds from the pastry. Spread the pastry with mustard, leaving a 1cm border around the edge.

3 Combine the broccoli, vegetarian cheddar, and mozzarella in a large bowl; season with salt and pepper. Place one-sixth of the broccoli mixture in the centre of a pastry round; fold over to enclose the filling, crimping the edge to seal. Repeat with the remaining broccoli mixture and pastry rounds.

4 Place the pies on trays. Brush with egg and sprinkle with the seeds; cut four slashes on each pie.

5 Bake the pies for 25 minutes or until golden and puffed.

Kale and walnut tarts

LACTO-OVO VEGETARIAN | PREP + COOK TIME **1 HOUR 20 MINUTES** | SERVES **6**

LSA mix consists of ground linseed, sunflower seeds, and almonds. It can be sprinkled on cereal, chopped fruit, and yogurt or used to enhance the health properties of smoothies and baked goods. It is a fantastic source of vitamins, minerals, fibre, and essential omega 3 oils.

40g butter, melted

2$\frac{1}{2}$ cups (310g) LSA (see tip)

2 eggs

30g baby kale leaves, finely chopped

$\frac{1}{3}$ cup roasted walnuts, chopped

$\frac{2}{3}$ cup (160g) ricotta, crumbled

4 eggs, extra

1$\frac{1}{3}$ cups (330ml) milk

2 tsp finely grated lemon rind

2 garlic cloves, crushed

2 tsp finely chopped fresh tarragon

salt and freshly ground black pepper

60g snow pea tendrils (pea shoots)

1 tbsp lemon juice

1 tbsp olive oil

1 Preheat oven to 200°C (180°C fan/400°F/Gas 6). Brush six 10cm loose-based fluted tart tins with half the melted butter. Place the tins on an oven tray.

2 Combine the LSA, eggs, and remaining melted butter in a medium bowl; season with salt and pepper. Press LSA mixture onto the bottoms and sides of the tins. Bake for 10 minutes; set aside to cool. Reduce oven to 160°C (140°C fan/325°F/Gas 3).

3 Divide the kale, walnuts, and ricotta between the tart cases. Whisk the extra eggs, milk, lemon rind, garlic, and tarragon in a large jug until combined; season with salt and pepper. Pour the egg mixture over the filling.

4 Bake the tarts for 30 minutes or until just set. Leave the tarts in tins for 5 minutes to cool slightly, but remove them from the tins while still warm (to prevent them from sticking).

5 Meanwhile, combine the snow pea tendrils, lemon juice, and olive oil in a small bowl; season with salt and pepper.

6 Serve the tarts topped with snow pea tendrils.

TIP

LSA mix can be found in some health food stores or purchased online. Alternatively, you can easily make your own version by blending 3 parts linseed, 2 parts sunflower seeds, and 1 part almonds until finely ground.

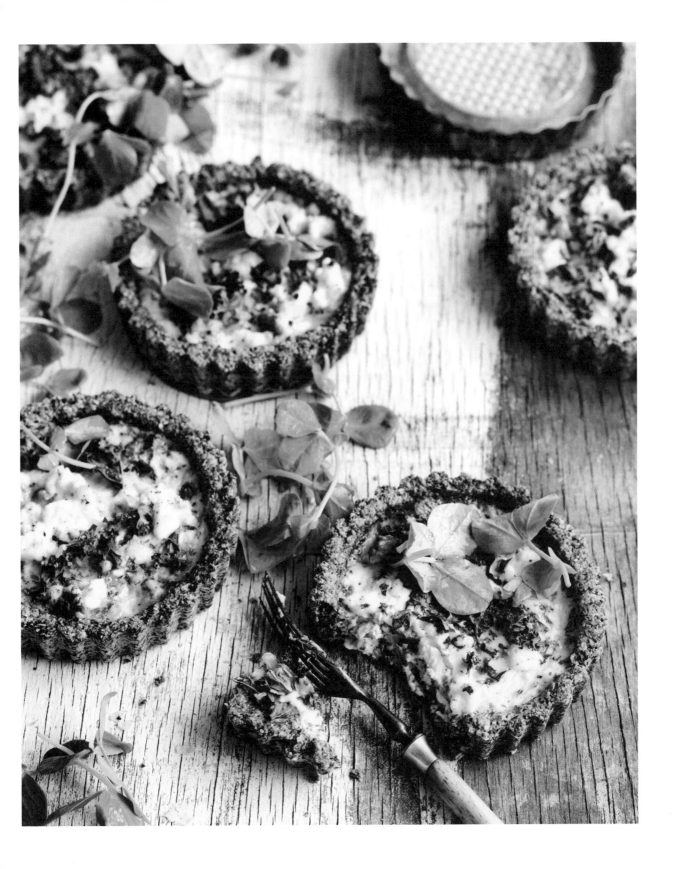

Kale

LACTO VEGETARIAN AND VEGAN

Kale is considered a superfood as it's such a great source of vitamins and minerals. In fact kale is one of the most nutrient-dense foods on the planet. It also possesses phytonutrients, which quell inflammation and can even protect brain cells from the effects of stress.

Smashed potatoes and kale

LACTO VEGETARIAN | PREP + COOK TIME **30 MINUTES** | SERVES **4**

Place 400g baby potatoes (halve any if large) and 1/2 teaspoon ground turmeric in a medium saucepan with enough cold water to cover; bring to the boil. Cook for 15 minutes or until tender. Drain. Heat 2 tablespoons of olive oil and 60g butter in the same pan; cook 1 crushed garlic clove and 400g torn kale leaves for 5 minutes or until the kale is wilted. Return the potatoes to the pan, using the back of a spoon, lightly smash each potato. Add 2 tablespoons each of dukkah and mint leaves; toss to combine.

Red rice and kale salad

LACTO VEGETARIAN | PREP + COOK TIME **50 MINUTES** | SERVES **2**

Preheat oven to 200°C (180°C fan/400°F/Gas 6). Cook 1 cup (200g) red rice in a medium saucepan of boiling water for 35 minutes. Add 1 cup (240g) frozen peas and 250g coarsely chopped green beans; cook for a further 5 minutes or until the rice and vegetables are tender; drain. Rinse under cold water; drain. Meanwhile, toss 150g purple kale with 2 tablespoons of olive oil on a baking-paper-lined oven tray; season with salt and pepper. Roast for 10 minutes or until crisp. Whisk 1 1/2 teaspoons of Dijon mustard, 1 tablespoon of white wine vinegar, and 2 1/2 tablespoons of olive oil in a small bowl; season. Combine the rice mixture, half the kale, and dressing. Serve the salad topped with the remaining kale and 100g crumbled feta.

Raw kale and broccoli salad

VEGAN | PREP TIME **20 MINUTES** | SERVES **2**

Coarsely chop 2 cups (70g) of firmly packed purple kale leaves. Discard the large thick stem from a 350g whole broccoli; cut into medium-sized florets. Quarter and core 1 medium (230g) pear. Using a mandoline or V-slicer, cut the broccoli florets and pear quarters into thin slices. Arrange the kale, broccoli, and pear on a serving platter. Combine 2 teaspoons of tamarind puree, 2 tablespoons of tamari, 1 tablespoon of lime juice, 2 teaspoons of sesame oil and 2 tablespoons of sesame seeds in a jug; drizzle over the salad.

Kale and walnut pesto

LACTO VEGETARIAN | PREP + COOK TIME **20 MINUTES** | SERVES **4**

Process 2 cups (70g) kale with 1/2 cup (10g) fresh flat-leaf parsley, 1 cup (80g) finely grated parmesan, 1/4 cup (60ml) lemon juice, 2 tablespoons of roasted walnuts, and 1 cup (250ml) extra virgin olive oil until almost smooth. Season with salt and pepper. Cook 400g wholemeal spaghetti or short tubular pasta in a saucepan of boiling salted water until almost tender; drain, reserving 1/4 cup (60ml) of the cooking liquid. Return pasta to the pan, off the heat. Add the pesto and reserved cooking liquid; toss gently until combined. Serve topped with chilli flakes.

CLOCKWISE from top left

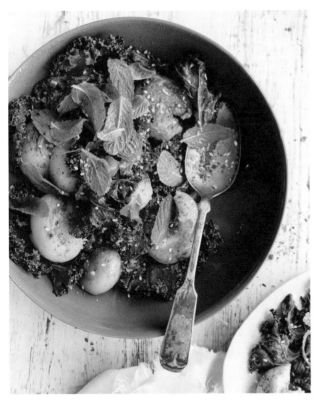
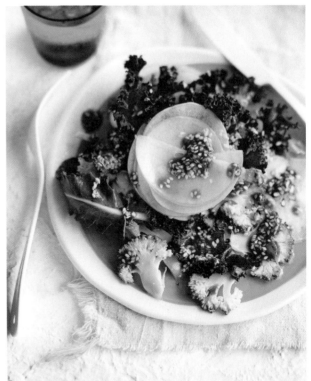
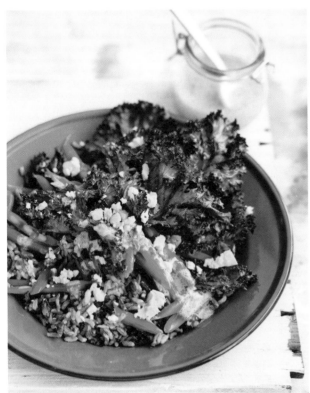
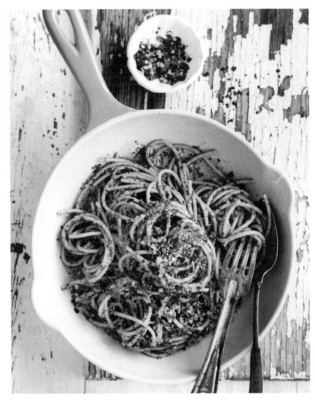

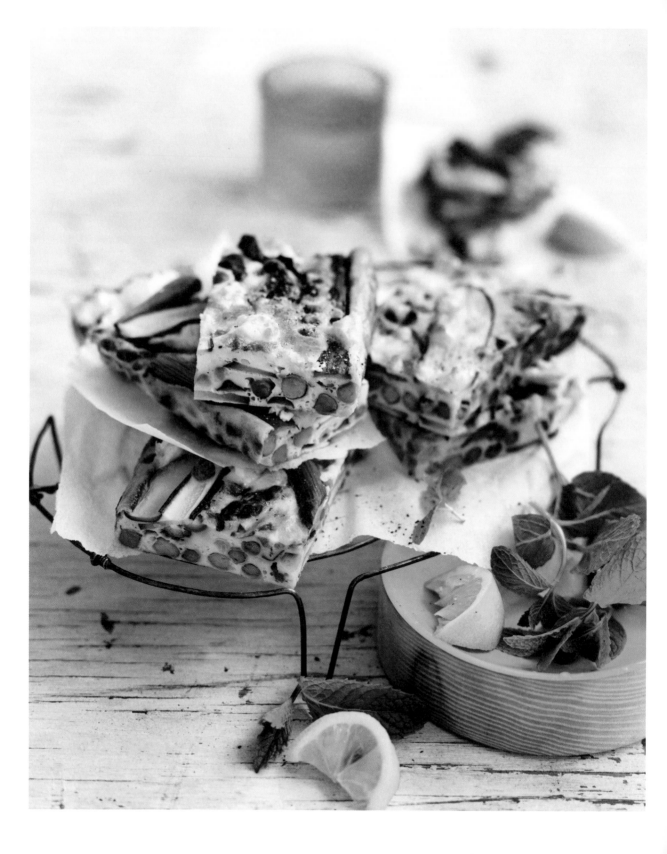

Asparagus and feta frittata

LACTO-OVO VEGETARIAN | PREP + COOK TIME **35 MINUTES + COOLING** | SERVES **6**

A frittata is Italy's version of an omlette; egg-based and laden with any number of ingredients. Feta and glorious greens star in this fresh tasting, nutrition-packed veggie version that's perfect for serving on its own or as part of a tapas lunch.

170g asparagus, trimmed, coarsely chopped

2 small courgettes (180g), thinly sliced lengthways

1 cup (120g) frozen peas

150g feta, crumbled

8 eggs

½ cup (125ml) single cream

½ cup (4g) fresh mint leaves, torn

salt and freshly ground black pepper

lemon wedges, to serve (optional)

1   Preheat oven to 180°C (160°C fan/350°F/Gas 4). Oil a 20cm x 30cm rectangular pan; line the bottom and two sides with baking paper, extending the paper 5cm (2in) over the edge.

2   Place the asparagus, courgette, and peas in a small saucepan of boiling water. Return to the boil; drain. Refresh in a bowl of iced water until cold. Drain well; pat dry with paper towel. Place the vegetables in a pan with the feta.

3   Whisk the eggs and cream in a large jug until combined; add the mint and season with salt and pepper. Pour the mixture over the vegetables.

4   Bake the frittata for 25 minutes or until set. Cool before cutting into pieces. Serve with lemon wedges, if you like.

TIP

The frittata can be eaten warm or at room temperature. Store cooled frittata, covered, in the fridge for up to 2 days.

Roasted garlicky pumpkin and sage pies

LACTO-OVO VEGETARIAN | PREP + COOK TIME **1 HOUR 30 MINUTES + REFRIGERATION** | MAKES **6**

These autumnal pumpkin and sage pies with a delicious spiced pastry crust make either a wonderful light lunch or starter. For bite-sized pies to serve as finger food at a party, you could make these in a couple of mini-muffin trays.

900g butternut pumpkin (butternut squash), chopped

4 garlic cloves, unpeeled

1 tbsp olive oil

3 eggs, lightly beaten

$1/2$ cup (125ml) single cream

$1/4$ cup (3g) coarsely chopped fresh sage

salt and freshly ground black pepper

75g feta, crumbled

$1^1/_2$ tbsp pepitas (pumpkin seeds), toasted

spicy pastry

$1^1/_2$ cups (225g) plain flour

1 tsp ground coriander

1 tsp cumin seeds

125g cold butter, coarsely chopped

1 free-range egg yolk

2 tbsp iced water, approximately

1   Preheat oven to 220°C (200°C fan/425°F/Gas 7).

2   Place the pumpkin and garlic on a baking-paper-lined oven tray, drizzle with oil. Bake for 20 minutes or until tender. Transfer to a large bowl; cool for 5 minutes. Squeeze the garlic from skins. Mash the pumpkin and garlic coarsely with a fork. Stir in the eggs, cream, and sage; season with salt and pepper.

3   Meanwhile, to make the spicy pastry, process the flour, spices, and butter until crumbly. Add the egg yolk and most of the water; process until the ingredients just come together. Enclose the pastry in plastic wrap (cling film); refrigerate for 30 minutes.

4   Grease six 9cm x 12cm oval or round pie tins. Divide the pastry into six even pieces. Roll each piece between sheets of baking paper until large enough to line the tins. Lift the pastry into the tins; press into the sides, trim the edges. Refrigerate for 20 minutes.

5   Reduce oven to 200°C (180°C fan/400°F/Gas 6). Place the tins on an oven tray; cover the pastry with baking paper, fill with dried beans or rice. Bake for 10 minutes. Remove the paper and beans; bake for a further 5 minutes or until lightly browned. Cool

6   Fill the pastry cases with the pumpkin mixture; sprinkle with feta. Bake for 35 minutes or until set and browned. Serve the pies topped with the pepitas.

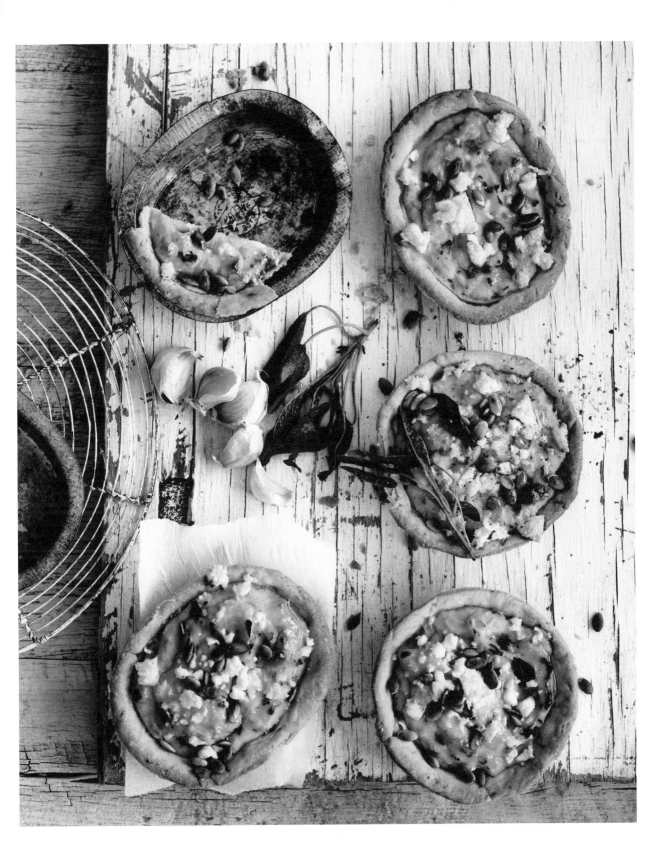

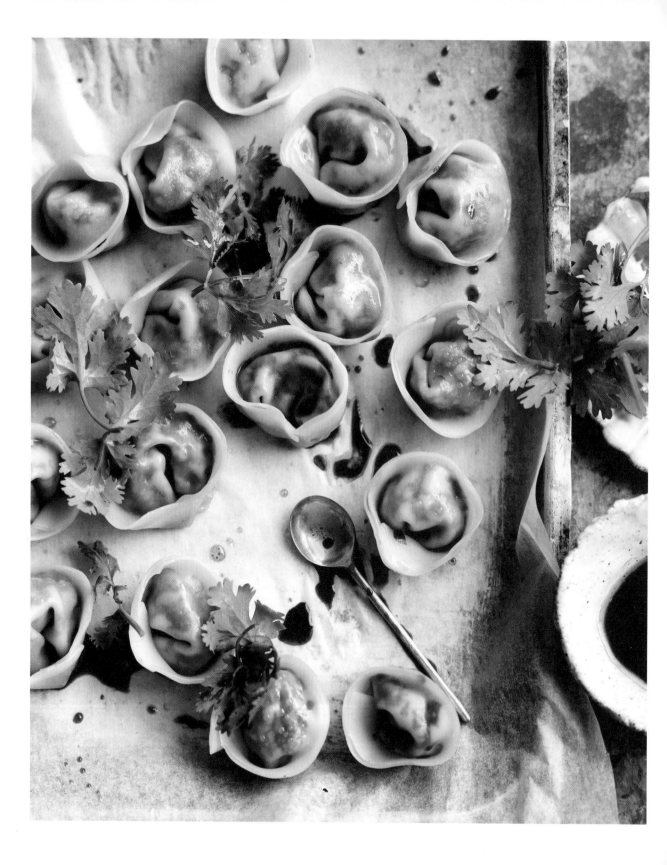

Green dumplings with soy chilli sauce

VEGAN | PREP + COOK TIME **45 MINUTES** | SERVES **4**

These freshly steamed dumplings are pure comfort food, Asian style. The wonton shape
of these nutritious parcels is similar to Italian tortellino and they are often boiled in a
light broth to make a dumpling soup.

300g spinach, trimmed

125g gai lan leaves (Chinese broccoli)

1 cup (60g) fresh finely chopped garlic chives

2 tbsp soy sauce

2 garlic cloves, finely grated

1½ tbsp finely grated fresh ginger

2 tsp sesame oil

240g round gow gee (wonton) wrappers

soy chilli dipping sauce

¼ cup (60ml) soy sauce

2 tbsp chinese black vinegar

1 tsp caster sugar

1 tsp sesame oil

1 tsp chilli oil

1 green onion (spring onion), thinly sliced

1   Boil, steam, or microwave the spinach and gai lan until tender; drain.
    Rinse under cold water; drain. Squeeze out excess water; chop finely.

2   Combine the spinach, gai lan, chives, soy sauce, garlic, ginger, and
    sesame oil in a medium bowl.

3   Place 2 teaspoons of the mixture in the centre of a gow gee wrapper.
    Wet the edge of the wrapper with your fingers; fold in half and press the
    edges together to seal. Repeat with the remaining wrappers and mixture.

4   Cook the dumplings, in batches, in a large saucepan of boiling water, for
    2 minutes, or until they float and are just tender. Drain.

5   Meanwhile, to make the soy chilli dipping sauce, combine the ingredients
    in a small bowl.

6   Serve the dumplings with the dipping sauce.

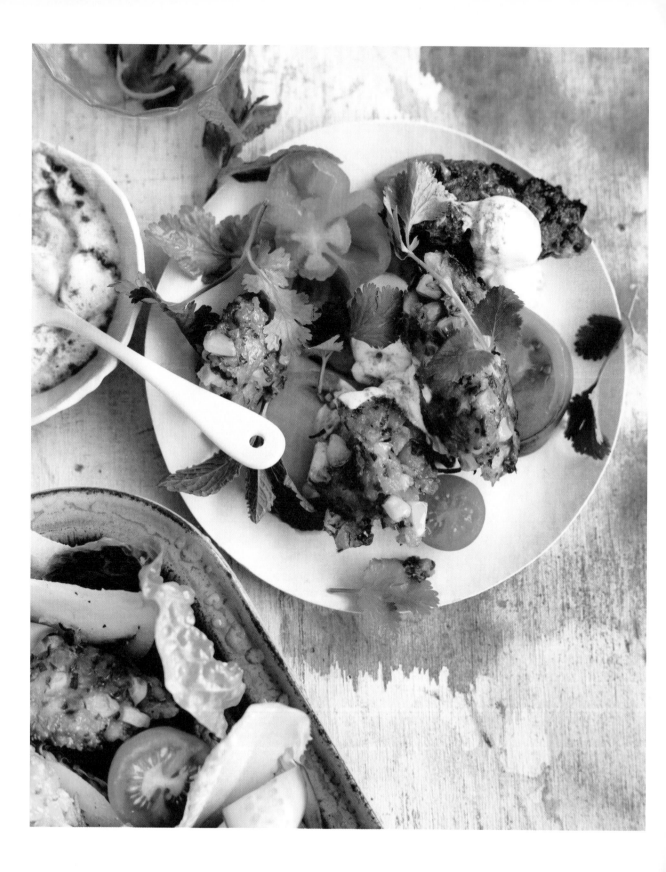

Corn and chickpea kofta with harissa yogurt

LACTO-OVO VEGETARIAN | PREP + COOK TIME **45 MINUTES** | SERVES **4**

Popular in the Middle East, koftas are traditionally made with spiced meat. This veggie variation instead uses protein-rich chickpeas and corn. You could use Lebanese bread to wrap these up, with or without the lettuce.

2 corn cobs (800g), trimmed, husks and silks removed

1/2 cup (60ml) olive oil

salt and freshly ground black pepper

1 small brown onion (80g), finely chopped

3 tsp Moroccan seasoning (Ras El Hanout)

2 x 400g can chickpeas, drained, rinsed

1 free-range egg, lightly beaten

1/4 cup (35g) plain flour

1/4 cup (8g) finely chopped fresh coriander

1/4 cup (12g) finely chopped fresh mint

16 baby cos (romaine) lettuce leaves

1 cucumber (130g), peeled lengthways into ribbons

200g tomato medley, halved

harissa yogurt

1 cup (280g) Greek yogurt

2 tsp harissa paste

1 tsp honey

1/2 tsp ground cumin

1 Brush the corn with a little of the olive oil; season with salt and pepper. Cook the corn cobs on a heated oiled grill plate (or barbecue) over a medium heat, turning occasionally, for 15 minutes or until charred and tender. When cool enough to handle, cut the kernels from the cobs; place in a large bowl.

2 Meanwhile, preheat oven to 200°C (180°C fan/400°F/Gas 6).

3 Heat 2 teaspoons of the oil in a small frying pan over a medium heat; cook the onion, stirring occasionally, for 5 minutes or until soft. Add Moroccan seasoning; cook, stirring, for 1 minute or until fragrant. Transfer the mixture to the bowl with the corn; add the chickpeas, then mash coarsely. Stir in the egg, flour, and herbs; season with salt and pepper. Shape the mixture into 16 koftas; place on an oven tray.

4 Heat the remaining oil in the same pan; cook the koftas, in batches, over a medium heat, turning occasionally, for 5 minutes or until golden. Transfer to a lightly oiled oven tray. Bake for 10 minutes or until cooked through.

5 To make the harissa yogurt, combine the ingredients in a small bowl; season with salt and pepper to taste.

6 Serve the koftas in lettuce leaves with cucumber and tomato, drizzled with the harissa yogurt.

TIP

Koftas can be made a day ahead; reheat, covered in foil, in the oven.

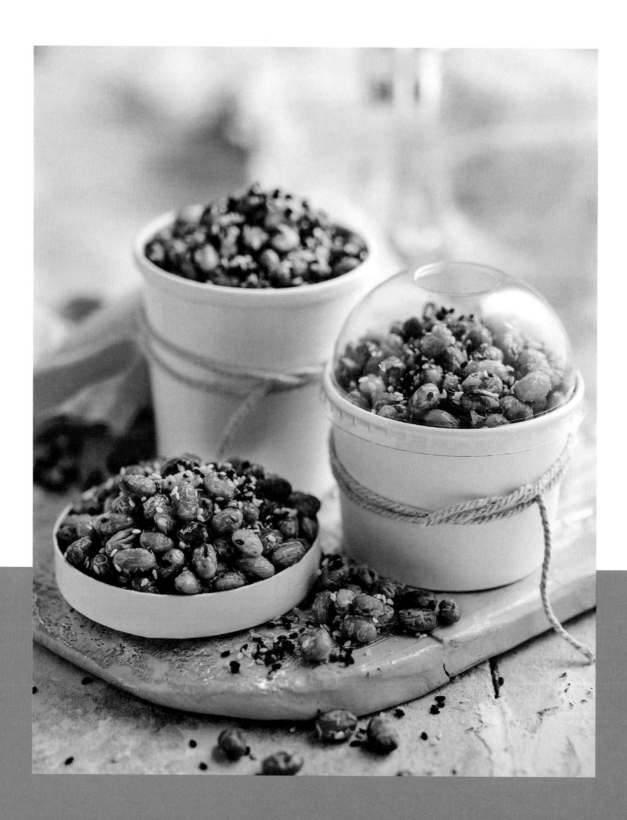

SNACKS AND SMALL BITES

Here you'll find an inspiring array of
alternative savoury snacks for healthy eating
on the go, plus a selection of small dishes
ideal for canapés and dinner party nibbles.

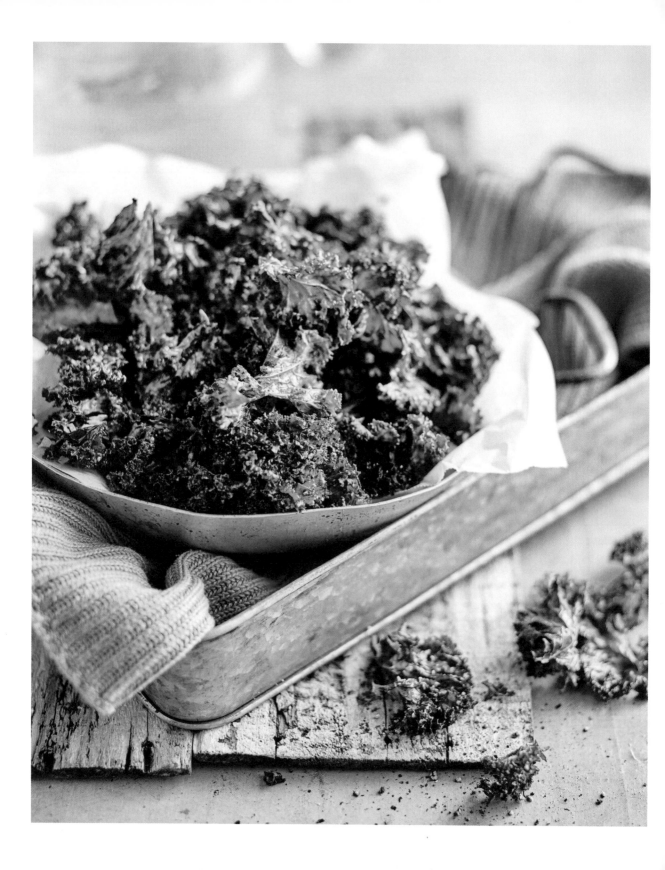

Kale chips

VEGAN | PREP + COOK TIME **25 MINUTES + COOLING** | SERVES **8**

These crunchy kale chips are as addictive as the potato variety, but with only a fraction of the calories and a far higher nutritional value. Great for serving at parties and as a healthy alternative for savoury snack lovers.

450g kale

1 tbsp extra virgin olive oil

1/2 tsp crushed sea salt flakes

1 Preheat oven to 190°C (170°C fan/375°F/Gas 5); place three large oven trays in the oven while preheating.

2 Remove and discard the kale stems from the leaves. Wash the leaves well; pat dry with paper towel or in a salad spinner. Tear the kale leaves into 5cm pieces; place in a large bowl, then drizzle with olive oil and sprinkle with salt. Using your hands, rub the oil and salt through the kale. Spread the coated kale, in a single layer, on trays.

3 Bake the kale for 10 minutes. Remove any pieces of kale that are already crisp. Return the remaining kale to the oven for a further 2 minutes; remove any pieces that are crisp. Repeat until all the kale is crisp. Cool.

TIP

These kale chips will keep in an airtight container for up to 2 weeks.

Roasted mixed olives and feta

LACTO VEGETARIAN | PREP + COOK TIME **25 MINUTES** | SERVES **6**

Bring a taste of the Mediterranean to your table with these fragrant, zingy roasted olives.
These make an easy yet delicious canapé or dinner party nibble. Use pitted olives,
if you prefer.

1 tsp each fennel seeds, cumin seeds,
and coriander seeds

1 medium lemon (140g)

300g mixed olives

1 tsp freshly ground black pepper

1/4 cup (60ml) olive oil

2 tbsp sherry vinegar

2 garlic cloves, thinly sliced

1 fresh long red chilli, thinly sliced

200g firm feta, cut into cubes

3 fresh thyme sprigs

1 Preheat oven to 180°C/350°F. Line an oven tray with baking paper.

2 Lightly crush the seeds with a mortar and pestle. Dry-fry the crushed seeds in a small frying pan over a medium heat, shaking the pan frequently, for 1 minute or until fragrant.

3 Using a vegetable peeler; peel rind from the lemon, avoiding any white pith. Cut the rind into long thin strips.

4 Combine the olives, lemon rind, pepper, olive oil, vinegar, garlic, chilli, feta, thyme, and toasted crushed seeds in a medium bowl. Arrange the olive mixture on the oven tray.

5 Bake for 8 minutes or until hot. Serve warm.

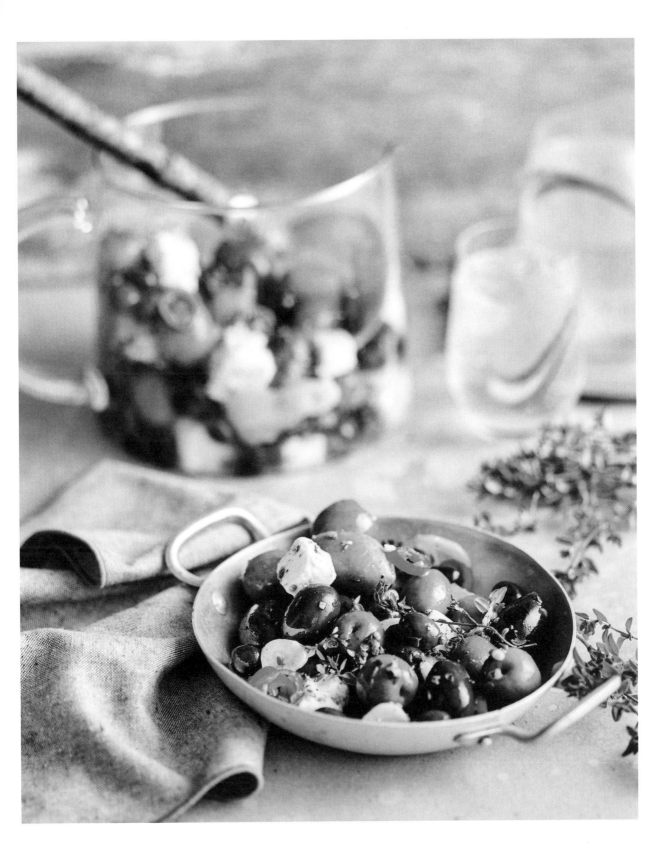

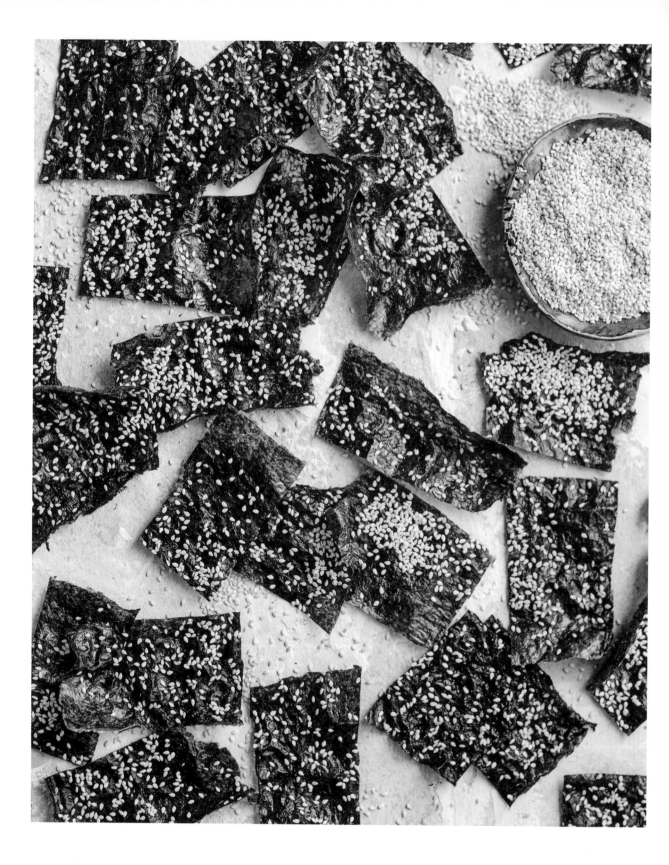

Nori sesame chips

VEGAN | PREP + COOK TIME **20 MINUTES** | MAKES **60 PIECES**

Nori is the Japanese name for dried edible seaweed sheets, best known for its use in making sushi. With a high nutritional value these nori chips are a great alternative to potato chips or other heavily salted snacks. To make this recipe gluten-free swap the soy sauce for tamari.

10 yaki nori sheets (25g)

1¹/₂ tbsp salt-reduced soy sauce

2¹/₂ tsp sesame oil

1¹/₂ tbsp white sesame seeds

1 Preheat oven to 150°C/300°F. Line three large oven trays with baking paper.

2 Place two sheets of nori, shiny-side up, on each tray. (If two sheets don't fit on one tray, cook one at a time.)

3 Combine the soy sauce and sesame oil in a small bowl. Brush half the soy mixture on the nori sheets on trays; sprinkle with half the sesame seeds.

4 Bake the nori for 8 minutes or until crisp. Transfer to wire racks to cool.

5 Repeat with the remaining nori sheets, soy mixture, and sesame seeds, re-using the trays and baking paper.

6 Cut each sheet into six pieces before serving.

TIP

Keep nori chips in an airtight container for up to 2 weeks.

Parsnip hummus with spiced chickpeas

VEGAN | PREP + COOK TIME **1 HOUR 15 MINUTES** | SERVES **8**

This smooth, creamy hummus swaps chickpeas as the main ingredient for deliciously
sweet and earthy roasted parsnips. Served with crisp parsnip chips and spicy chickpeas
it's a showstopping snack.

4 medium parsnips (1kg), peeled, coarsely chopped

2 tbsp olive oil

salt and freshly ground black pepper

2 garlic cloves, crushed

2 tbsp tahini

$^3/_4$ cup (180ml) vegetable stock

$^2/_3$ cup (160ml) olive oil, extra

$1^1/_2$ tbsp apple cider vinegar

$^1/_4$ cup (5g) coarsely chopped fresh flat-leaf parsley

2 Lebanese flatbreads, toasted, torn into large pieces

parsnip chips

2 medium parsnips (500g), peeled

cooking-oil spray

spiced chickpeas

2 tbsp olive oil

2 medium red onions (340g), halved, thinly sliced

2 x 400g can chickpeas, drained, rinsed

2 garlic cloves, sliced

1 tbsp cumin seeds

2 tsp ground coriander

$^1/_2$ tsp chilli flakes

2 tbsp pomegranate molasses

1 Preheat oven to 180°C (160°C fan/350°F/Gas 4). Line a large oven tray with
baking paper. Combine the parsnip and olive oil on the tray. Season with
salt and pepper. Roast for 45 minutes or until tender; cool slightly.

2 Increase oven to 220°C (200°C fan/425°F/Gas 7). To make the parsnip
chips, line two large oven trays with baking paper. Using a vegetable
peeler, peel the parsnips into thin ribbons. Place on the trays; lightly
spray with cooking oil. Season with salt and pepper. Bake for 8 minutes,
turning halfway through cooking time, or until golden.

3 Process the roasted parsnips with the garlic, tahini, stock, extra oil,
and vinegar until the mixture is smooth. Season with salt and pepper
to taste.

4 To make the spiced chickpeas, heat the olive oil in a large frying pan over
a medium heat; cook the onion, stirring occasionally, for 8 minutes or
until soft. Add the chickpeas and the garlic; cook, stirring, for 3 minutes.
Stir in the spices and chilli; cook for 2 minutes. Stir in the pomegranate
molasses; season with salt.

5 Top the parsnip hummus with half the chickpeas and half the parsley.
Serve with the remaining chickpeas and parsley, as well as the flatbread
and parsnip chips.

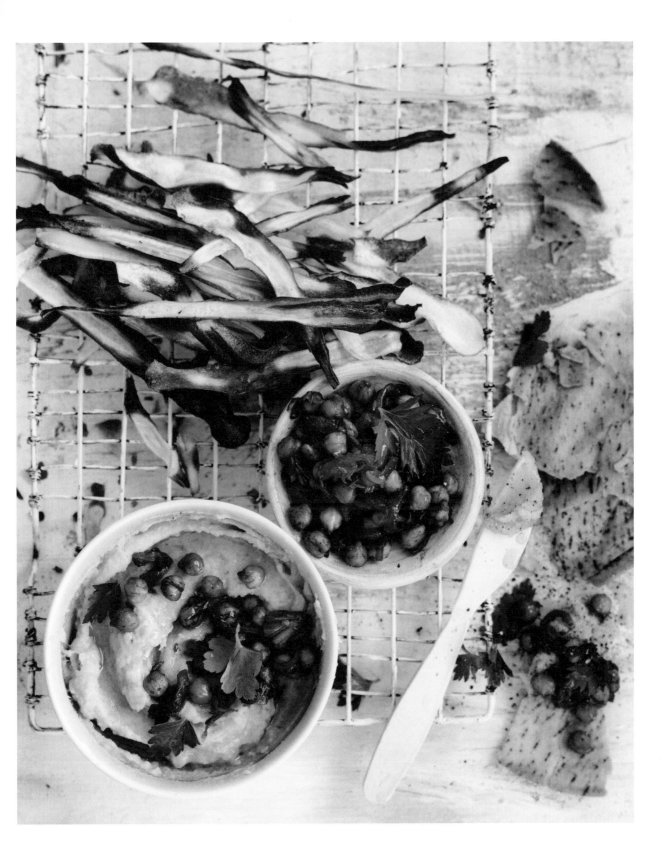

Cheese and kimchi toasties

LACTO VEGETARIAN | PREP + COOK TIME **1 HOUR + REFRIGERATION** | SERVES **6**

The homemade flatbreads in this recipe make these cheesy toasties something special –
perfect for supper or a scrumptious snack. For the kids, you can always leave out the kimchi
and use sliced tomato instead.

1¹/₄ cups (185g) plain flour

¹/₂ cup (75g) self-raising flour

pinch of bicarbonate of soda

2 tsp caster sugar

1 green onion (spring onion), thinly sliced

2 tsp black sesame seeds

2 tsp white sesame seeds

1 tsp sea salt flakes

1 tsp freshly ground black pepper

¹/₂ cup (140g) natural yogurt

¹/₃ cup (80ml) water

2 tbsp vegetable oil

1¹/₂ cups (150g) grated mozzarella

2 cups (450g) kimchi, drained

1¹/₂ cups (185g) grated gruyère cheese

1 cucumber (130g), cut into long thin ribbons

¹/₄ cup (4g) fresh coriander leaves

¹/₄ cup (2g) fresh mint leaves

1   Sift the flours, bicarbonate of soda, and sugar into a large bowl; stir in the green onion, seeds, salt, and pepper. Combine the yogurt, water, and half the oil in a jug. Pour the yogurt mixture into the dry ingredients; stir to combine. Knead the dough on a floured surface for 5 minutes or until smooth. Cover; refrigerate for 30 minutes.

2   Divide the dough into six portions. Roll each portion on a floured surface into oval shapes about 2mm thick and 25cm long. Brush the dough with the remaining oil; cook on a heated oiled grill plate (or grill or barbecue) for 2 minutes each side or until the flatbreads are golden and cooked through.

3   Place ¹/₄ cup (25g) of the mozzarella on one half of each flatbread; top each with ¹/₄ cup (60g) of the kimchi, then ¹/₄ cup (30g) of the gruyère. Fold the flatbread over the filling. Cook the flatbreads on a heated oiled grill plate for 1 minute each side or until the cheeses melt.

4   Serve the toasties warm with cucumber and herbs.

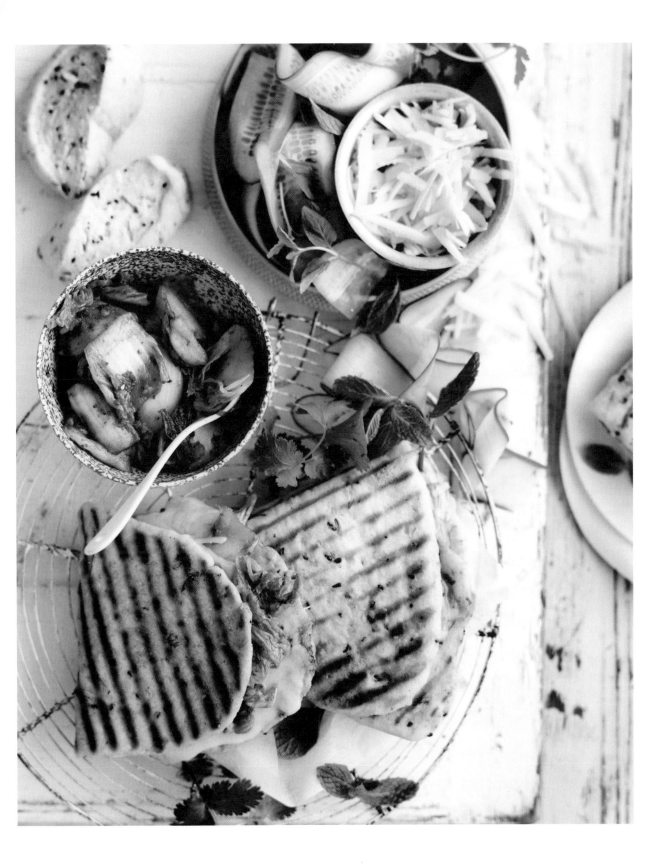

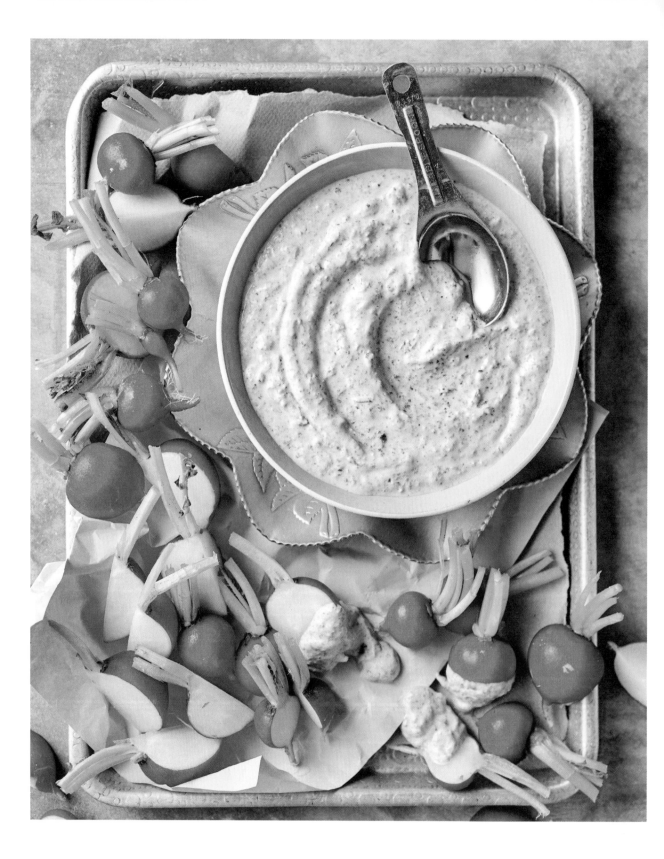

Spiced yogurt, cucumber, and herb dip

LACTO VEGETARIAN | PREP + COOK TIME **15 MINUTES** | MAKES **1½ CUPS (420g)**

This fragrant cooling raita-style sauce makes a great dip for raw vegetable crudités or can serve as a cool counterpoint to warm, spicy dishes. The dip is best made on the day of serving, but can be kept refrigerated for up to 3 days.

1 medium cucumber (130g)

1 tsp sea salt flakes

½ cup (8g) fresh coriander leaves

1 cup (8g) fresh mint leaves, extra

2 garlic cloves, crushed

1 fresh long green chilli, seeded, chopped coarsely

½ tsp ground cumin

1 cup (280g) Greek yogurt

500g red radishes, trimmed, large ones halved or quartered

1   Halve the cucumber lengthways; remove seeds. Coarsely grate the cucumber. Toss the cucumber and salt together in a medium bowl. Place in a sieve; stand for 5 minutes. Squeeze the cucumber with your hands to remove excess liquid. Transfer to a medium bowl.

2   Meanwhile, blend or process the herbs, garlic, chilli, cumin, and 1 tablespoon of the yogurt until smooth.

3   Add the herb mixture to the cucumber in the bowl with the remaining yogurt; stir until the dip mixture is well combined.

4   Serve the dip with radishes.

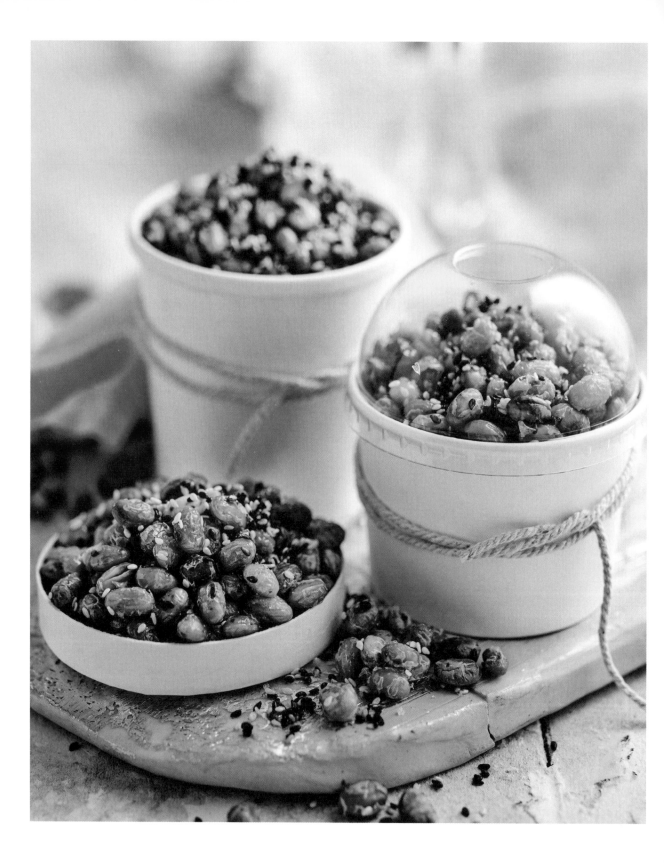

Roasted sesame edamame beans

VEGAN | PREP + COOK TIME **25 MINUTES** | SERVES **4**

Edamame beans are available shelled, in the pod, fresh, or frozen. They make a super-healthy snack, being naturally gluten-free and low in calories, and contain no cholesterol. In addition they are an excellent source of protein, iron, and calcium.

500g edamame beans, shelled (see tip)

2 tsp olive oil

2 tsp black sesame seeds

2 tsp white sesame seeds

½ tsp sesame oil

½ tsp salt flakes

1   Preheat oven to 220°C (200°C fan/425°F/Gas 7). Line an oven tray with baking paper.

2   Place the ingredients in a medium bowl; stir to combine. Spread the mixture onto the oven tray.

3   Bake for 15 minutes or until golden.

TIP

You can use fresh or frozen (thawed) edamame; available from Asian food stores and some supermarkets. To quickly thaw the beans, place in a heatproof bowl, top with hot water; stand for 1 minute. Drain, then shell.

Seed crackers with smashed avocado

VEGAN | PREP + COOK TIME **1 HOUR 30 MINUTES** | MAKES **50 CRACKERS**

Don't worry if there are holes when you roll out the crackers – these will give them texture and character. If you find it easier, you could leave the crackers as whole sheets and break into pieces after baking.

1 cup (200g) long-grain brown rice

2¹/₂ cups (625ml) water

1 cup (200g) tri-colour quinoa

2 cups (500ml) water, extra

¹/₄ cup (35g) sesame seeds

¹/₄ cup (50g) linseeds

¹/₄ cup (35g) chia seeds

¹/₄ cup (35g) sunflower seeds

1 tbsp finely chopped fresh lemon thyme

1 tbsp finely chopped fresh oregano

1 tbsp finely chopped fresh rosemary

1 tsp cracked black pepper

2 tsp onion powder

salt and freshly ground black pepper

1 medium avocado (250g)

1 tbsp lemon juice

2 tsp chia seeds, extra

45g snow pea shoots

pinch of sumac, optional

1 Preheat oven 180°C (160°C fan/350°F/Gas 4).

2 Place the brown rice and the water in a small saucepan; bring to the boil. Reduce heat to low; simmer, uncovered, for 25 minutes or until most of the water has evaporated. Remove from the heat; stand, covered, for 10 minutes. Fluff with a fork, spread out over an oven tray; cool.

3 Place the quinoa and the extra water in the same pan; bring to the boil. Reduce the heat to low; simmer, uncovered, for 10 minutes or until most of the water has evaporated. Remove from heat; stand, covered, for 10 minutes. Fluff with a fork, spread out over an oven tray; cool.

4 Process the rice with half the quinoa to form a coarse paste; transfer to a large bowl. Add the remaining quinoa, seeds, herbs, pepper, and onion powder. Season with salt and pepper. Using your hands, combine well. Divide into four portions.

5 Line four oven trays with baking paper. Remove one of the pieces of baking paper. Flatten a portion of dough over the paper, cover with plastic wrap (cling film) then roll out with a rolling pin to 1mm-thick. Discard the plastic; carefully lift the paper back onto the tray. Repeat with the remaining portions of dough until you have four trays. Score the crackers into 5cm x 10cm lengths or triangles.

6 Bake the crackers for 20 minutes. Cover the crackers with a sheet of baking paper and a second tray. Holding the hot tray with oven gloves, flip the crackers over onto the second tray; carefully remove lining paper. Repeat with the remaining trays. Cook the crackers for a further 20 minutes or until golden and crisp. Cool on trays.

7 To serve, roughly smash the avocado with a fork in a small bowl with the lemon juice; season with salt and pepper to taste. Place 4 crackers on each of the two serving plates; top the crackers with the avocado mixture, extra chia seeds, snow pea shoots, and sumac if using.

TIPS

• If the cracker mixture spreads past the paper when you're rolling it just cut those edges off.

• Crackers can be stored in an airtight container for up to 1 month.

144

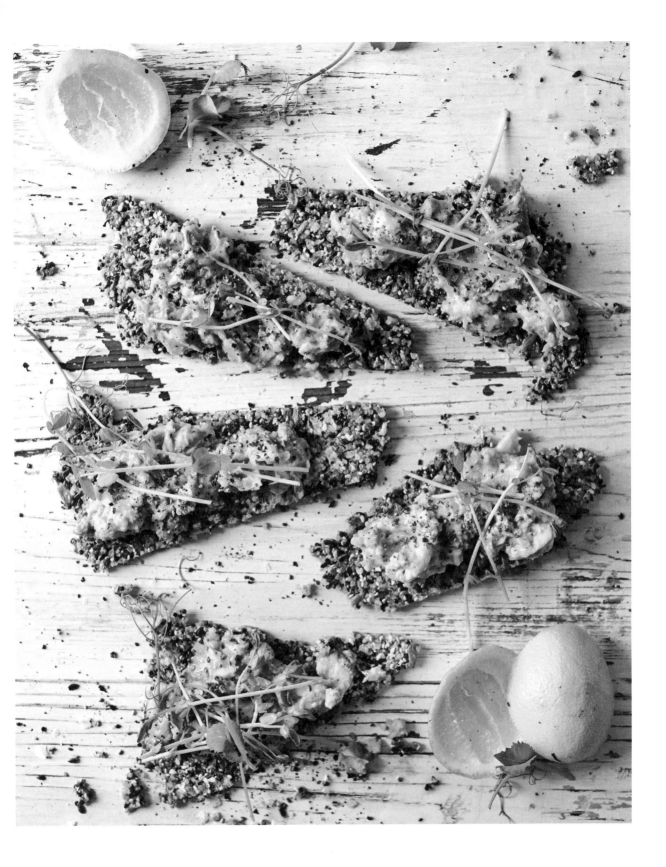

Chia and tomato guacamole with sumac crisps

VEGAN | PREP + COOK TIME **20 MINUTES** | SERVES **4**

Adding chia seeds to your guacamole gives it an extra kick of nutritious goodness. They may be small but these little wonders are an excellent source of omega-3 fatty acids and antioxidants, and they're brimming with fibre and protein.

cooking oil spray

4 rye flatbreads breads (100g)

1½ tsp ground sumac

salt and freshly ground black pepper

2 medium avocados (500g), coarsely chopped

⅓ cup (80ml) lime juice

1 small red onion (100g), finely chopped

⅓ cup (60g) semi-dried tomatoes, finely chopped

¼ cup (4g) fresh coriander, coarsely chopped

½ tsp smoked paprika

1½ tbsp black or white chia seeds

2 fresh long red chillies, sliced thinly

1 Preheat oven to 200°C (180°C fan/400°F/Gas 6). Line three oven trays with baking paper; spray with cooking oil.

2 Cut each sheet of flatbread into 16 triangles. Place in a single layer on the trays; spray with oil. Sprinkle with sumac; season with salt and pepper. Bake for 5 minutes or until golden and crisp.

3 Place the avocado and lime juice in a medium bowl; mash lightly with a fork. Stir in the red onion, tomato, coriander, paprika, 1 tablespoon of the chia seeds, and three-quarters of the chilli. Season to taste with salt.

4 Place the guacamole in a serving bowl; top with the remaining chilli and remaining chia seeds. Serve with the sumac crisps.

TIP

Guacamole can be stored, covered, in the fridge for up to 2 days. Sumac crisps will keep in an airtight container at room temperature for up to 1 week.

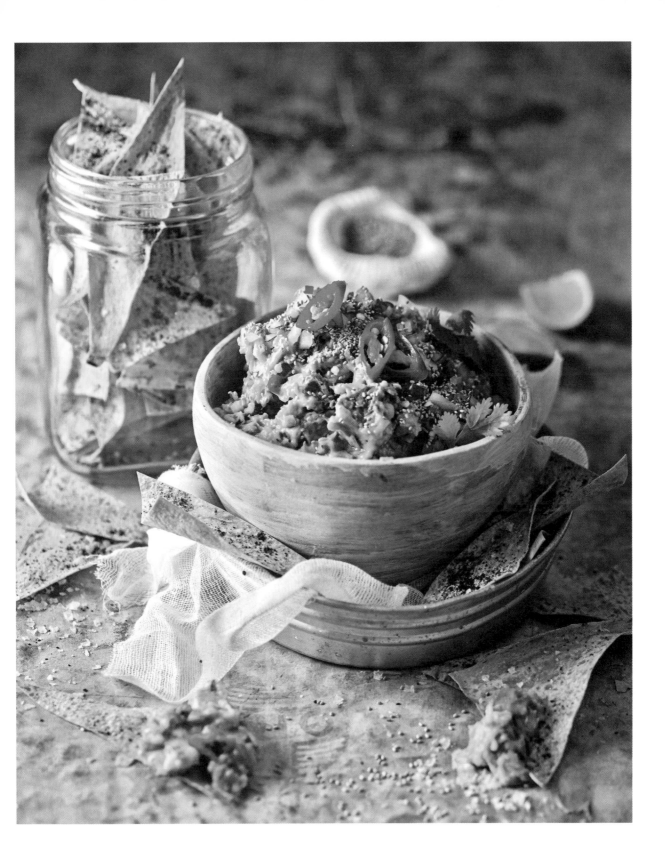

Vegan yogurt

VEGAN

You can experiment with different nuts to create this yogurt, bearing
in mind the flavour each nut will create. Stir in the juice of a lemon
for a great savoury yogurt option.

Basic vegan yogurt

PREP TIME **5 MINUTES + STANDING** | MAKES **2½ CUPS (625ML)**

Place 1 cup (150g) cashews and 1 cup (160g) whole blanched
almonds in a large bowl; cover with cold water. Stand, covered,
for 4 hours or overnight. Drain; rinse under cold water. Drain.
Process nuts with 1 cup (250ml) water until it forms a
yogurt-like consistency.

Strawberry yogurt

PREP TIME **10 MINUTES + STANDING** | MAKES **2½ CUPS (625ML)**

Make basic yogurt on left using 1 cup (150g) cashews and
1 cup (120g) pecans. Blend or process 250g strawberries until
smooth. Fold the strawberry puree through the yogurt to create
a swirled effect.

Passionfruit yogurt

PREP TIME **5 MINUTES + STANDING** | MAKES **2½ CUPS (625ML)**

Make basic yogurt on left; stir in the pulp of 3 passionfruit.

TIPS

- Store vegan yogurts in the fridge for up to 1 week.
- You could use blueberries or raspberries instead of
  strawberries, if you prefer.

CLOCKWISE from top

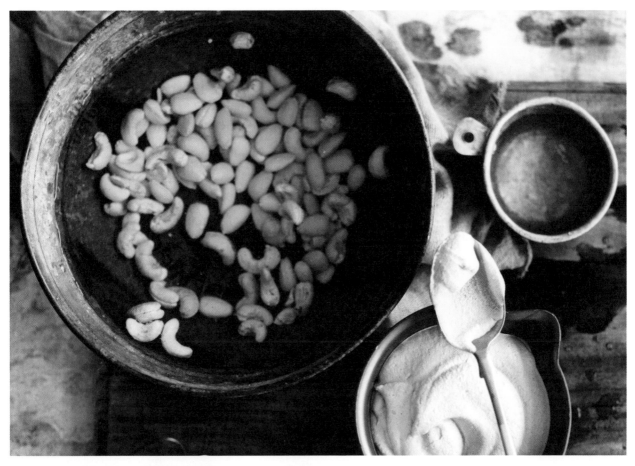

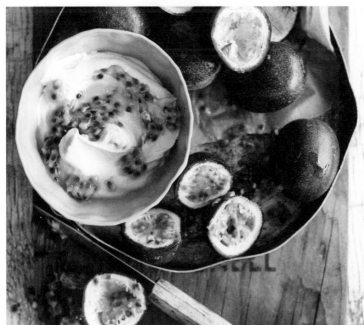

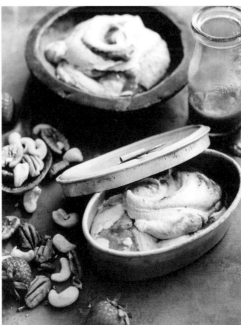

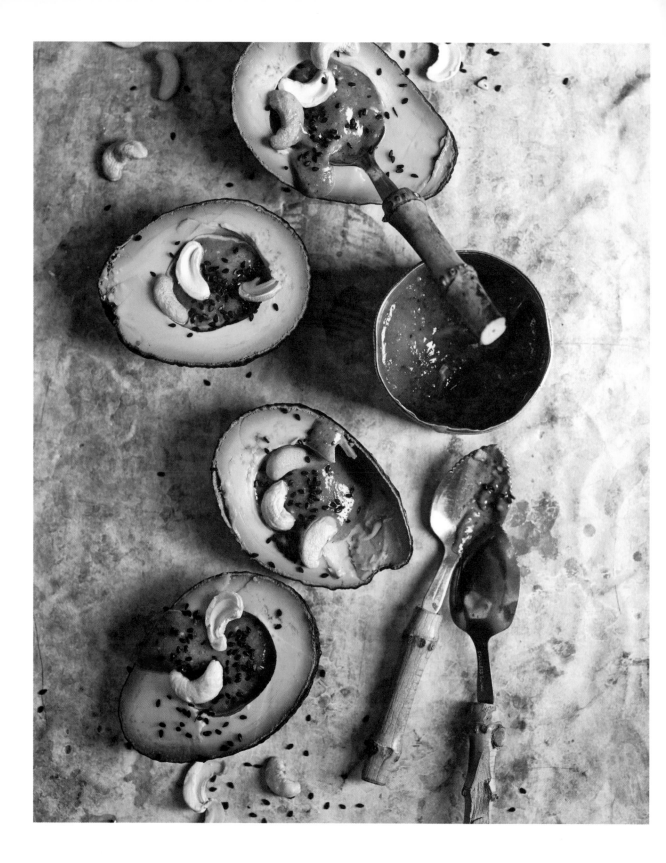

Miso almond butter with avocado

VEGAN | PREP + COOK TIME **15 MINUTES** | SERVES **4**

This versatile nutty butter can also be used as a dressing for salads or a dip for vegetables and is delicious melted over sweet potatoes or swirled into stir-fries. Keep it in an airtight container and use as desired.

1½ tbsp white (shiro) miso

2 tbsp almond butter

2 tbsp olive oil

½ tsp sesame oil

1 tbsp mirin

1 tbsp water

salt and freshly ground black pepper

2 medium avocados (500g)

⅓ cup (50g) roasted cashews, chopped coarsely

½ tsp black sesame seeds

1 Stir the miso, almond butter, oils, mirin, and water in a medium jug until smooth; season with salt and pepper to taste.

2 Cut the unpeeled avocados in half; discard stones. Spoon the dressing into the avocado hollows; sprinkle with cashews and sesame seeds. Serve immediately.

Roasted sweet and sour chickpeas and beans

VEGAN | PREP + COOK TIME **1 HOUR** | MAKES **2½ CUPS (300g)**

You can use dried legumes instead of the chickpeas and beans – soak them overnight first and cook for 1½ hours in boiling water. Experiment with different spices and herbs to flavour however you like.

2 x 400g can chickpeas

2 x 400g can butter beans

1 tbsp extra virgin olive oil

1 tbsp finely grated lime rind

2 tsp ground cumin

2 tsp ground coriander

1 tsp chilli flakes

1 tbsp coconut sugar

salt and freshly ground black pepper

1 Preheat oven to 220°C (200°C fan/425°F/Gas 7). Line an oven tray with baking paper.

2 Drain then rinse the chickpeas and butter beans; place in a medium heatproof bowl. Cover with boiling water; drain. Dry on paper towel. (This will ensure that the chickpeas and beans will dry and crisp up during roasting.)

3 Place the chickpeas and beans on the oven tray. Bake for 50 minutes, stirring occasionally, or until golden and crisp.

4 Transfer the roasted chickpeas and beans to a medium bowl. Add the olive oil, lime rind, cumin, coriander, chilli flakes, and coconut sugar. Season generously with salt and freshly ground black pepper; toss until well coated.

TIP

Store the roasted mix in an airtight container or jar for up to 4 days.

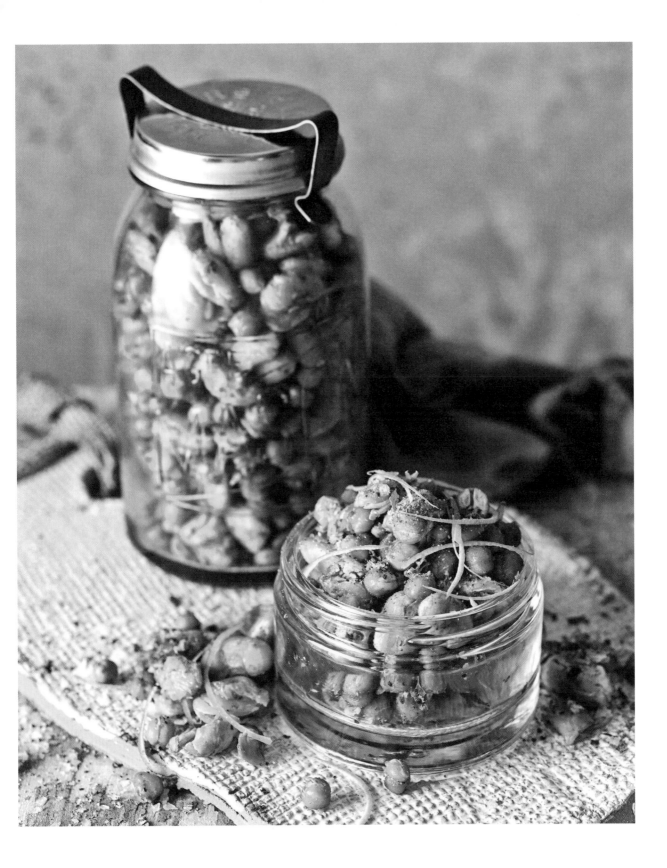

Cheese biscotti

LACTO-OVO VEGETARIAN | PREP + COOK TIME **1 HOUR 20 MINUTES + COOLING** | MAKES **20 PIECES**

These savoury biscotti are given added crunch and bite with the addition of nuts and spices. They should keep well in an airtight container for up to a week, but if they soften, return them to the oven to re-crisp. For a gluten-free option, use gluten-free self-raising flour instead.

1 cup (120g) almond meal (ground almonds)

½ cup (80g) wholemeal self-raising flour

2 tsp dried oregano leaves

½ tsp baking powder

¼ tsp cayenne pepper

½ cup (40g) finely grated vegetarian parmesan (make sure it doesn't contain animal rennet)

1 cup (120g) coarsely grated vegetarian cheddar

2 eggs

¼ cup (60ml) olive oil

1   Preheat oven to 180°C (160°C fan/350°F/Gas 4). Line an oven tray with baking paper.

2   Combine the almond meal, flour, oregano, baking powder, and cayenne pepper in a medium bowl. Add the vegetarian parmesan and vegetarian cheddar; mix well.

3   Whisk the eggs and olive oil in a small jug. Add the egg mixture to the cheese mixture. Using your hands, bring the mixture together. Turn the dough out onto a lightly floured surface. Shape, then roll the mixture into a 25cm log. Place the log on the oven tray; flatten slightly.

4   Bake for 35 minutes or until lightly browned. Leave on the tray for 15 minutes.

5   Reduce oven to 160°C (140°C fan/325°F/Gas 3).

6   Using a large serrated knife, cut the log diagonally, into 1cm slices. Place the slices, in a single layer, on an oven tray. Bake for 15 minutes. Turn the biscotti over. Bake for a further 12 minutes or until lightly browned. Cool on wire racks.

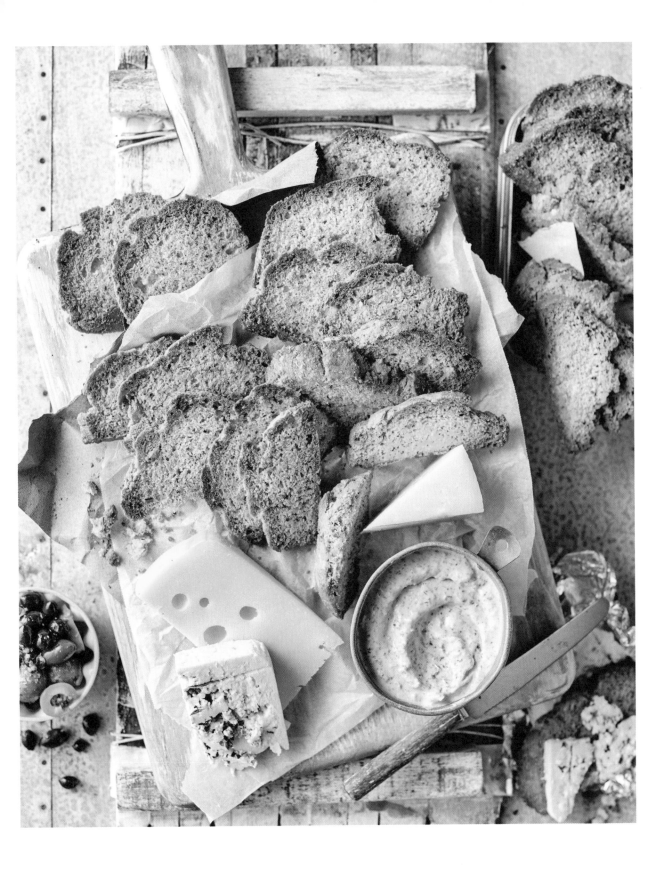

Cheesy cajun popcorn

LACTO VEGETARIAN | PREP + COOK TIME **10 MINUTES** | MAKES **7 CUPS (400g)**

Bring a little something extra to movie-night snacks with this addictive savoury popcorn that combines cheese with a twist of cajun spiciness. The cooled popcorn will keep in an airtight container for up to three days.

1 tbsp olive oil

25g butter

¼ cup (60g) popping corn

2 tsp Cajun seasoning mix

2 tsp salt flakes

½ cup (40g) finely grated vegetarian parmesan

1 Heat the olive oil and butter in a medium saucepan over a medium-high heat until starting to bubble.

2 Add the popping corn, seasoning mix, and salt; cover the pan with a tight fitting lid. Cook, shaking the pan occasionally, for 3–5 minutes or until the popping has stopped.

3 Remove pan from the heat. Add the vegetarian parmesan to the popcorn; stir until well coated.

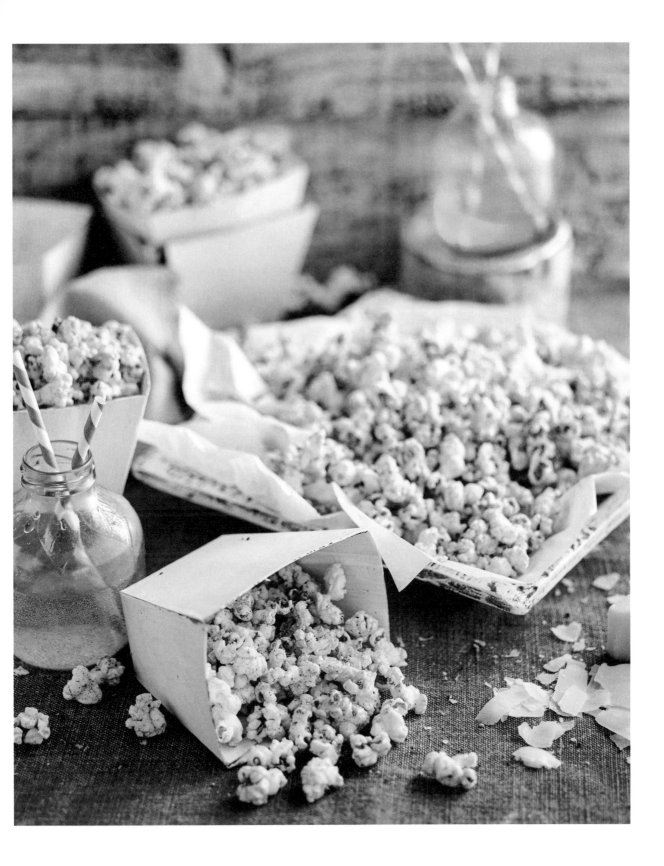

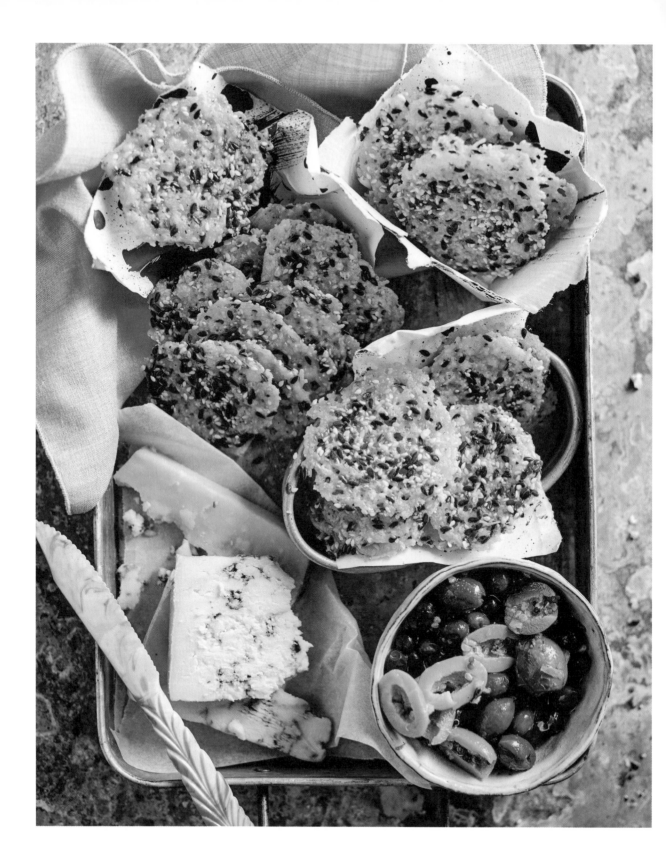

Seeded vegetarian parmesan crisps

LACTO VEGETARIAN | PREP + COOK TIME **30 MINUTES** | MAKES **24**

These parmesan crisps are so simple to make and are a great alternative savoury snack.
Serve with cheese and olives or munch on them unadorned. They also work well crumbled
over salads instead of croutons. Store in an airtight container for up to a week.

2 cups (160g) finely grated vegetarian parmesan
(make sure it doesn't contain animal rennet)

1 tbsp white chia seeds

1 tbsp linseeds

1 tbsp white sesame seeds

Freshly ground black pepper

1 Preheat oven to 180°C (160°C fan/350°F/Gas 4). Line two large oven trays
with baking paper.

2 Place level tablespoons of vegetarian parmesan in mounds on trays.
Flatten mounds to about 7.5cm across, leaving 2.5cm between rounds.
Combine the seeds in a small bowl; sprinkle half a teaspoon of seed
mixture on each round. Season lightly with freshly ground black pepper.

3 Bake the crisps for 12 minutes or until melted and lightly golden. Cool on
trays. Transfer to an airtight container.

Dukkah spiced trail mix

OVO VEGETARIAN | PREP + COOK TIME **35 MINUTES + COOLING** | MAKES **4 CUPS**

Trail mix consists of a mixture of dried fruit and nuts and was designed to be eaten as a snack on hikes. Lightweight and easy to carry, it's great for providing a quick energy boost during or after exercise. This version is livened up by the addition of the spice blend, dukkah.

1 cup (140g) roasted salted peanuts

1 cup (160g) natural almonds

1/2 cup (70g) whole skinless hazelnuts

1/2 cup (100g) pepitas (pumpkin seeds)

1 cup (50g) flaked coconut

2 free-range egg whites, lightly beaten

45g dukkah

1/2 tsp table salt

1/4 cup (40g) dried currants

1 Preheat oven to 180°C (160°C fan/350°F/Gas 4). Line two oven trays with baking paper.

2 Combine the nuts, pepitas, and coconut in a large bowl.

3 Combine the egg white, dukkah, and salt in a small bowl; add to the nut mixture. Stir until well combined. Divide the mixture between the trays in a single layer.

4 Bake for 10 minutes. Sprinkle each with currants; bake for a further 8-10 minutes or until lightly browned and fragrant. Cool on trays.

5 Separate the trail mix into small clusters. Store in an airtight container.

TIP

Trail mix can be kept in an airtight container at room temperature for up to 2 weeks.

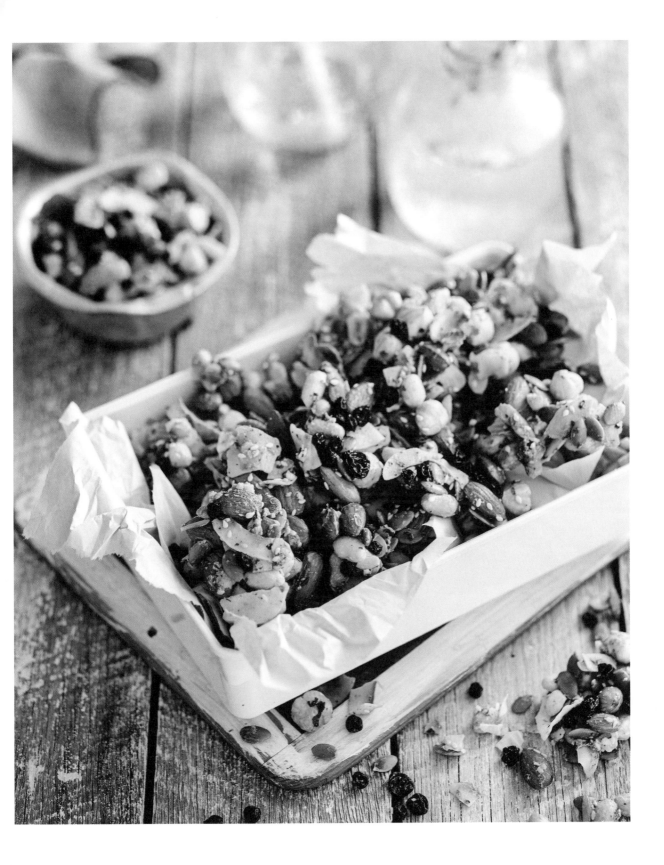

Vegetable bean curd rolls

VEGAN | PREP + COOK TIME **45 MINUTES** | SERVES **4**

Bean curd sheets are available from Asian food stores. If they are hard to find, you could
use fresh rice noodle sheets or blanched cabbage leaves instead. Steam
as the recipe directs.

50g dried rice vermicelli noodles

1 tbsp sesame oil

200g shiitake mushrooms, thinly sliced

100g enoki mushrooms, trimmed

3 cups finely shredded wombok cabbage
(Chinese leaf)

200g green beans, thinly sliced

1 medium carrot (120g), cut into matchsticks

1 cup (80g) bean sprouts

1/3 cup (80ml) char siu sauce

2 tbsp tamari or soy sauce

2 tbsp toasted sesame seeds

4 bean curd sheets (125g)

1 tsp cornflour

1 Place the noodles in a small heatproof bowl, cover with boiling water,
stand until just tender; drain.

2 Heat the sesame oil in a wok over a high heat; stir-fry the mushrooms for
2 minutes or until golden and tender. Add the cabbage, beans, and
carrot; stir-fry for 1 minute or until almost tender. Add the bean sprouts,
noodles, 2 tablespoons of the char siu sauce, half the tamari, and half
the sesame seeds; stir-fry for 30 seconds or until heated through. Drain,
reserving the cooking liquid.

3 Halve the bean curd sheets. Top with the vegetable mixture. Fold the
sheet over the filling, then fold in both sides. Continue rolling to enclose
the filling. Repeat with the remaining vegetable mixture and sheets to
make a total of eight rolls.

4 Steam the rolls, covered, over a large wok of simmering water for
10 minutes or until the bean curd is tender.

5 Meanwhile, whisk the cornflour and reserved cooking liquid in a small
saucepan until combined. Stir in the remaining char siu sauce, tamari,
and sesame seeds. Place the pan over a medium-high heat; cook for 5
minutes or until the mixture boils and thickens.

6 Serve the vegetable rolls with sauce; sprinkle with extra sesame seeds,
if you like.

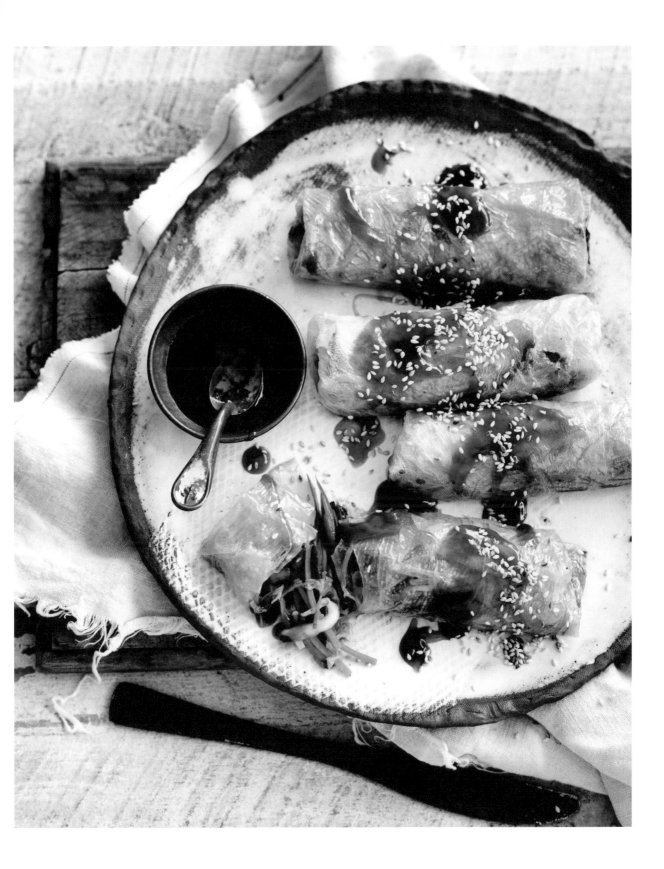

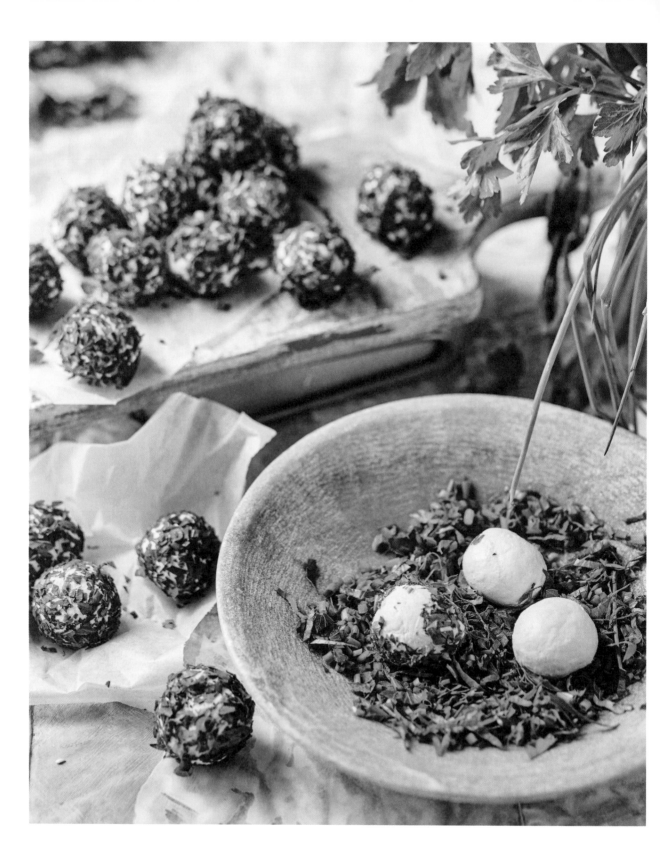

Cheese and herb balls

LACTO VEGETARIAN | PREP + COOK TIME **20 MINUTES + REFRIGERATION** | MAKES **12 BALLS**

Two types of cheese are simply rolled into balls and covered in herbs in this easy-to-make delicious cold appetiser or snack. Mild and creamy with added green freshness these are perfect for nibbles at a party or anytime snacking.

125g cream cheese, at room temperature

75g fresh goat's cheese, at room temperature

$1/3$ cup (7g) finely chopped fresh flat-leaf parsley

1 tbsp finely chopped fresh chives

1 Combine the cheeses in a medium bowl.

2 Roll 2 level teaspoons of the mixture into balls. Roll the balls in the combined herbs. Place the balls on a baking-paper-lined oven tray. Refrigerate for 1 hour.

TIP

These cheese balls can be stored in an airtight container in the refrigerator for up to 1 week.

Brown rice energy balls

VEGAN | PREP + COOK TIME **1 HOUR + REFRIGERATION** | MAKES **12**

Turn these energy balls into lunch, by stuffing them into a pita pocket or wrap along with salad ingredients and a little dressing made from Greek yogurt, a couple of teaspoons of tahini, and lemon juice.

1 cup (200g) medium-grain brown rice

2¹/₂ cups (625ml) vegetable stock

2 tbsp tahini

1 tbsp tamari

1 tbsp apple cider vinegar

2 tbsp chia seeds

2 green onions (spring onions), finely chopped

2 tsp finely grated fresh ginger

salt and freshly ground black pepper

2 tbsp black sesame seeds

2 tbsp white sesame seeds

1 Rinse the rice under running water until the water runs clear. Place the rice in a medium saucepan with the stock; bring to the boil. Reduce the heat to low; cook, covered, for 40 minutes or until the stock is almost absorbed and the rice is tender. Remove from the heat; stand, covered, for 5 minutes.

2 Transfer the hot rice to a medium bowl; immediately stir in the tahini, tamari, vinegar, chia seeds, green onion, and ginger. Season with salt and pepper to taste. Stand for 5 minutes or until cool enough to handle.

3 Roll 2 tablespoons of the mixture into balls; roll in the combined sesame seeds. Place the balls on a baking-paper-lined tray. Refrigerate for at least 30 minutes before eating.

TIP

Ingredients containing rice should always be kept refrigerated and never left at room temperature, otherwise food poisoning can occur. Rice balls will keep refrigerated for up to five days.

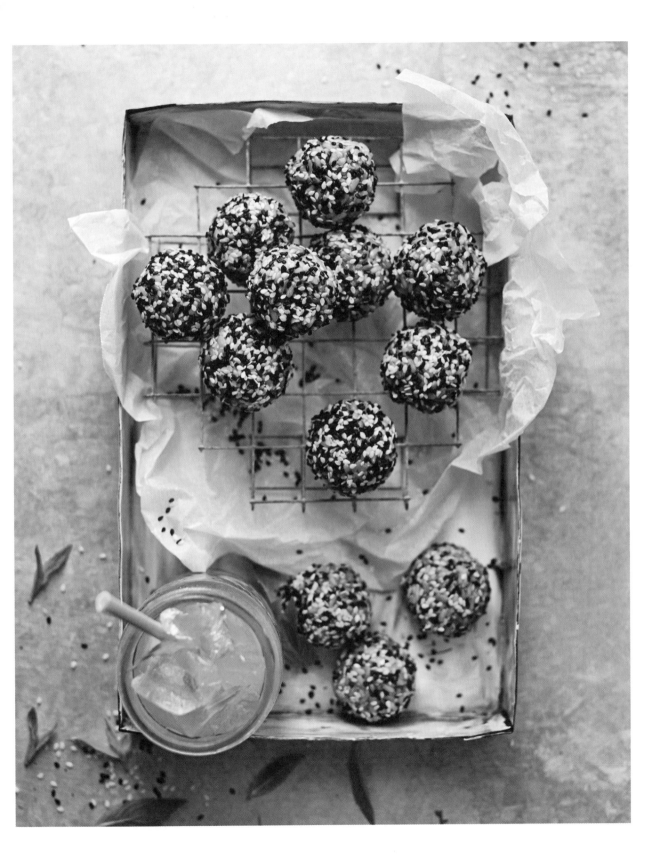

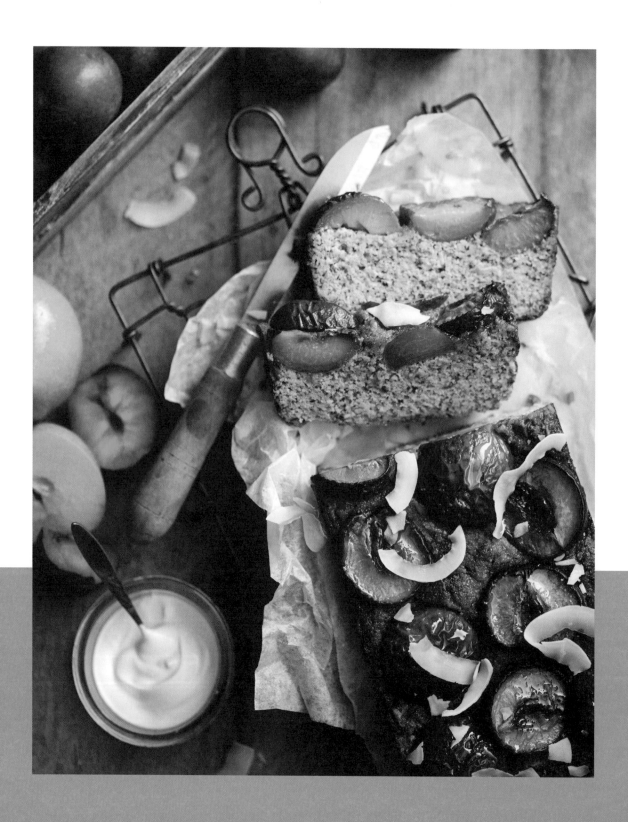

DESSERTS

From baked ricotta pudding through to
vegan cheesecake and mouthwatering white
chocolate blondies, these are decadent
desserts with a difference.

Pear and chocolate rye bread pudding

LACTO-OVO VEGETARIAN | PREP + COOK TIME **1 HOUR 20 MINUTES** | SERVES **4**

The sweetness of this creamy, rich pudding really enhances the tangy depth of the rye bread.
An ingredient not usually associated with desserts, the rye bread here makes a great contrast
to the sweet pears and rich chocolate.

300g loaf rye bread, torn into pieces

8 small paradise pears (450g), unpeeled, halved,
quartered, and some left whole

40g butter, softened

100g dark chocolate (70% cocoa), coarsely chopped

2 cups (500ml) milk

300ml pouring (single) cream

¼ cup (60ml) pure maple syrup

¾ tsp ground cinnamon

pinch of salt

3 eggs

2 tbsp pure maple syrup, extra

1   Preheat oven to 160°C (140°C fan/325°F/Gas 3). Grease a shallow 8-cup (2-litre) ovenproof dish.

2   Place the torn bread and pear in the dish, dot with butter then scatter with the chocolate.

3   Bring the milk, cream, maple syrup, cinnamon, and salt to the boil in a medium saucepan. Whisk the eggs in a large heatproof bowl. Gradually whisk the hot milk mixture into the egg. Pour the mixture over the bread mixture.

4   Bake the pudding for 50 minutes or until just set. Stand for 5 minutes before serving, drizzled with extra maple syrup.

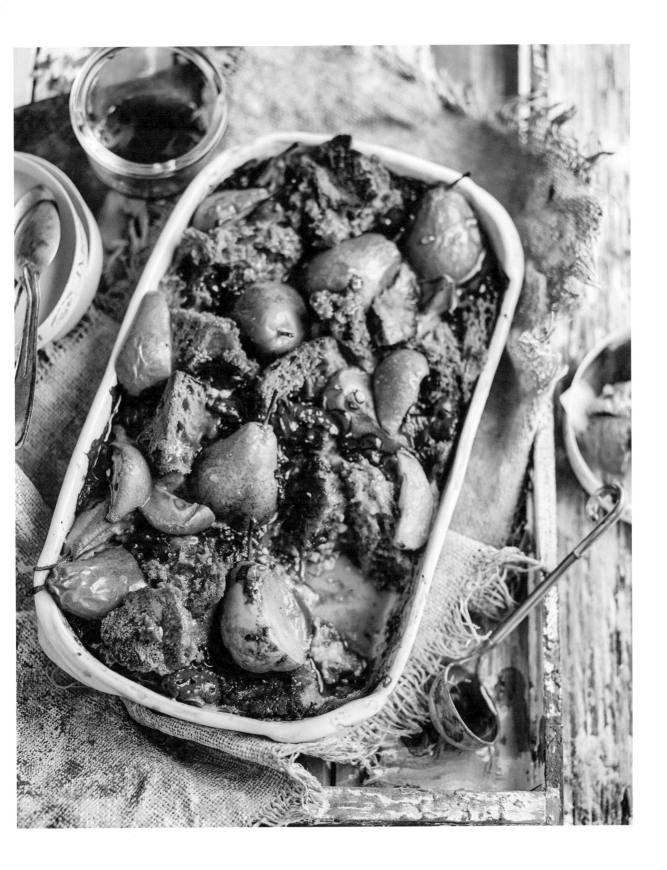

Raspberry ripple sweet corn ice-cream

VEGAN | PREP + COOK TIME **1 HOUR 30 MINUTES + STANDING & FREEZING** | MAKES **1 LITRE**

This healthy non-dairy ice-cream is made with corn, which provides a natural creaminess and sweetness. Expect the ice-cream to be slightly icier as a result. You could freeze the ice-cream mixture into blocks and roll in the cornflake crunch before serving.

2 trimmed corn cobs (500g)

2¼ cups (560ml) coconut cream

2 cups (500ml) unsweetened almond milk

¼ cup (55g) caster sugar

2 tsp vanilla extract

½ cup (125ml) agave syrup

1½ cups (225g) fresh or thawed frozen raspberries

cornflake crunch

2 tbsp caster sugar

1 tbsp agave syrup

1 tbsp olive oil

½ tsp vanilla extract

2 cups (80g) cornflakes

1 Using a sharp knife, cut the kernels from the cobs; reserve cobs. Place the corn kernels, cobs, coconut cream, almond milk, and sugar in a large saucepan over a medium-high heat; bring to the boil. Reduce heat; simmer for 5 minutes or until the corn is tender. Stand for 1 hour.

2 Discard the corn cobs. Blend or process the corn mixture until smooth. Strain the corn mixture; discard the solids. Stir in the vanilla and ⅓ cup (80g) of the agave syrup until combined.

3 Transfer the corn mixture to an ice-cream machine (see tip). Churn mixture following the manufacturer's instructions.

4 Meanwhile, blend or process the raspberries with the remaining agave syrup until smooth. Swirl the raspberry mixture through almost frozen ice-cream to create a ripple effect; pour into a 4-cup (1-litre) freezer-proof container. Freeze overnight or until firm.

5 Make the cornflake crunch. Preheat oven to 150°C (130°C fan/300°F/Gas 2). Line an oven tray with baking paper. Place the sugar, agave syrup, olive oil, and vanilla in a small saucepan over a low heat, stirring, until the sugar dissolves. Place the cornflakes in a medium bowl. Add the syrup mixture; stir to combine. Spread the cornflake mixture on the oven tray. Bake for 25 minutes or until slightly more golden. Leave to cool. Break into small pieces.

6 Serve the ice-cream topped with cornflake crunch.

TIP

If you don't have an ice-cream machine, place corn mixture only in the loaf pan, then cover with foil; freeze for 1 hour or until half frozen. Pulse mixture in a food processor to break-up ice crystals. Return to pan, cover with foil; repeat freezing and processing. Fold through the raspberry mixture, return to pan and cover with foil; freeze for 5 hours or overnight until frozen.

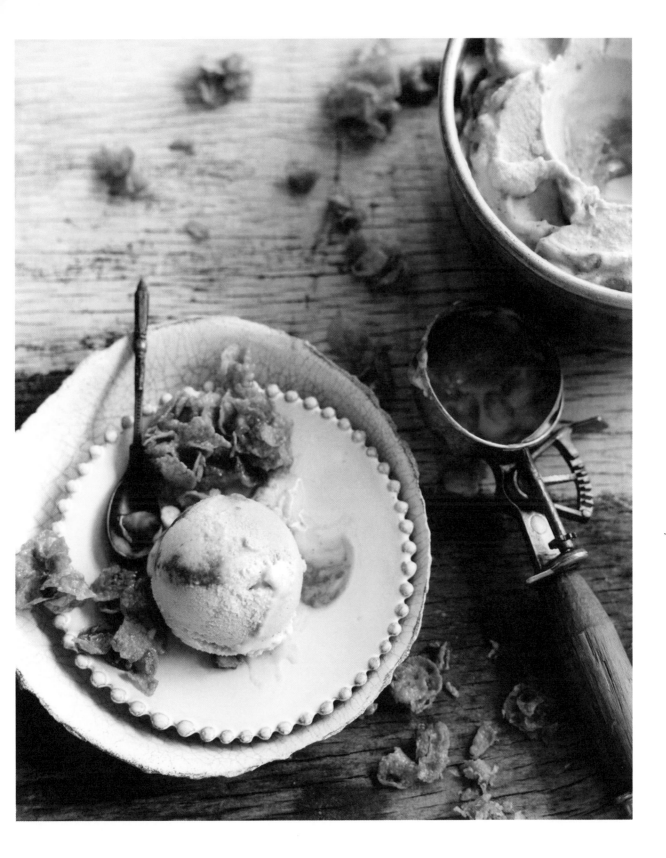

Earl grey and chocolate vegan cheesecake

VEGAN | PREP + COOK TIME **20 MINUTES + STANDING & REFRIGERATION** | SERVES **10**

This vegan cheesecake contains no cheese and is instead based on nuts, which bring added nutrients and a natural richness. When figs are not in season, serve the cheesecake topped with fresh raspberries and flaked almonds. You need to start this recipe the day before.

4 cups (600g) raw unsalted cashews

8 Earl Grey tea bags

¼ cup (25g) cacao powder

1 cup (230g) fresh dates, pitted

1 cup (200g) virgin coconut oil

2 tsp vanilla extract

8 small figs (400g), torn in half

2 tsp cacao powder, extra

cheesecake base

1 cup (170g) activated buckinis (buckwheat groats) (see tips)

½ cup (80g) natural almonds

⅓ cup (35g) cacao powder

1 cup (230g) fresh dates, pitted

¼ cup (50g) virgin coconut oil

2 tbsp warm water

1 tsp vanilla extract

1 Place the cashews and tea bags in a large bowl, cover with cold water; stand for 24 hours.

2 Grease a 22cm (9in) (base measurement) springform pan; line with baking paper.

3 Make the cheesecake base. Process the buckinis, nuts, and cacao powder until finely ground. With the motor operating, add the dates, coconut oil, water, and vanilla; process until well combined and the mixture sticks together when pressed.

4 Using the back of a spoon, spread the mixture evenly onto the bottom of the pan. Refrigerate for 15 minutes or until firm.

5 Drain the cashews and tea bags, reserving ½ cup (125ml) of the soaking liquid. Place the cashews in the bowl of a food processor; empty the tea leaves from the tea bags onto the cashews. Add the reserved soaking liquid, cacao, dates, coconut oil, and vanilla; process until the mixture is as smooth as possible. Spread the filling mixture over the chilled base. Refrigerate for at least 4 hours or until firm.

6 Before serving, top the cheesecake with figs and dust with extra cacao.

TIPS

- Activated buckinis are buckwheat groats that have been soaked, washed, rinsed, and dehydrated. The process is said to aid digestion.
- If you have one, use a high-powered blender when making the filling, to make the mixture very smooth.

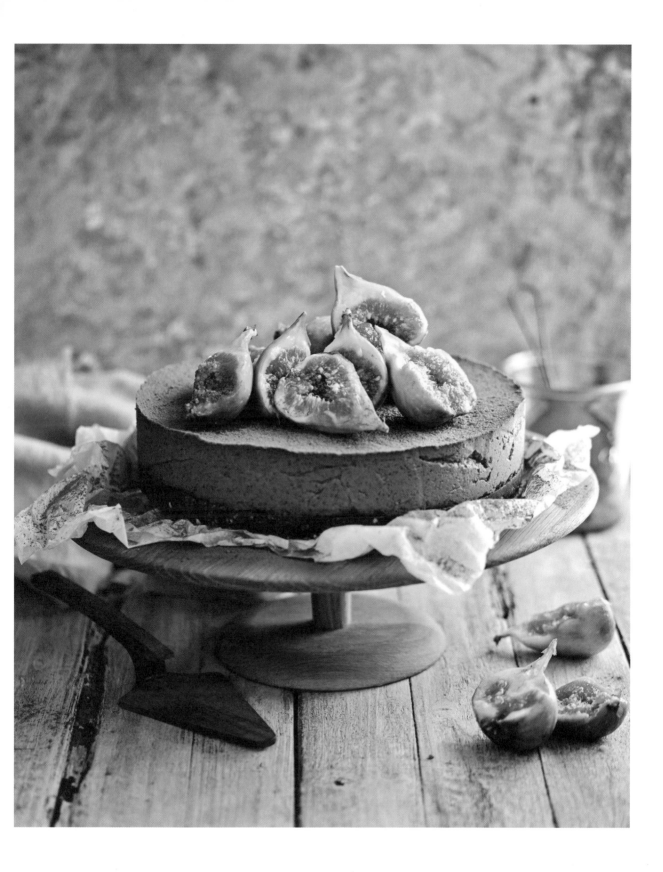

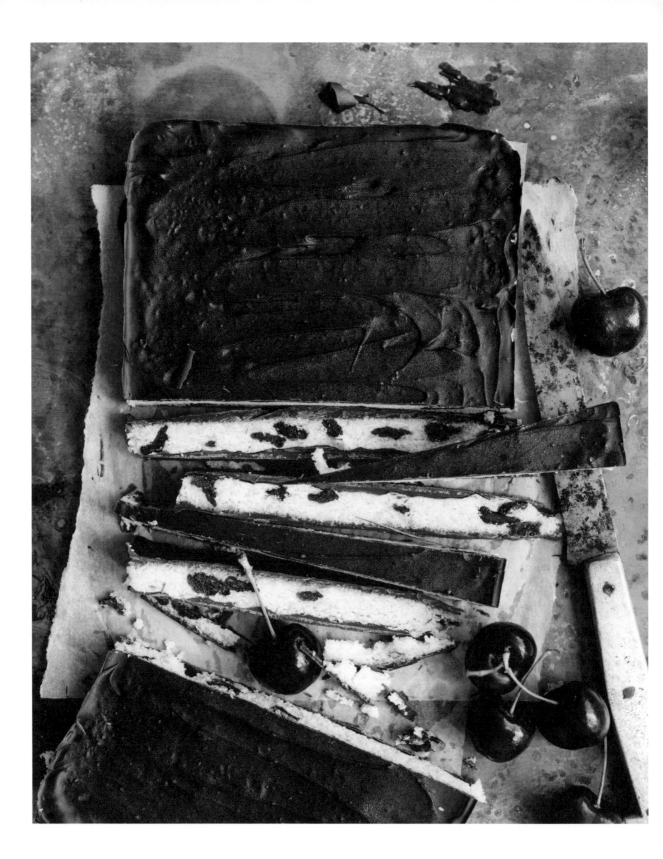

Choc-cherry coconut bars

VEGAN | PREP + COOK TIME **30 MINUTES + REFRIGERATION & FREEZING** | MAKES **16**

The vegan chocolate used in these no-bake bars is uncompromising in its flavour and packed with antioxidants. This delicious trio of chocolate, cherry, and coconut combines to make a moreish bar great for snacking or a lunchbox treat.

200g dark (semi-sweet) vegan chocolate, coarsely chopped (see tip)

1 cup (150g) dried cherries, finely chopped

3 cups (240g) desiccated coconut

1/2 cup (125ml) rice malt syrup

1 tsp vanilla extract

1/3 cup (80ml) melted coconut oil

1 Line the bottom and sides of an 18cm x 28cm slice pan with baking paper.

2 Place half the chocolate in a small heatproof bowl over a saucepan of gently simmering water (don't allow the bowl to touch the water); stir until just melted. Pour the chocolate into the pan; spread to cover the bottom. Refrigerate for 15 minutes or until set. Keep the water at a gentle simmer; reserve the bowl off the heat.

3 Combine the cherries and coconut in a large bowl; stir in the syrup, vanilla, and coconut oil until combined. Press the mixture very firmly in an even layer over the chocolate.

4 Return the pan of water to a gentle simmer over a medium heat. Place the remaining chocolate in the reserved bowl over the water; stir until melted. Pour the chocolate over the cherry coconut layer; spread evenly with a spatula. Freeze for 1 hour or until set (alternatively, refrigerate for 3 hours or until set). Cut into bars before serving.

TIP

Vegan chocolate is available at health food stores and some supermarkets.

Nut milks

VEGAN

You can make nut milks with most nuts: hazelnuts, almonds, cashews, pecans. If you want to sweeten the milk, add pure maple syrup, honey, or pureed dates.

Basic nut milk

PREP TIME **10 MINUTES + STANDING** | MAKES **2 CUPS (500ML)**

Place 1 cup (140g) skinless hazelnuts in a large bowl; cover with cold water. Stand, covered, for 4 hours or overnight. Drain; rinse under cold water. Drain. Process the nuts with 2 cups (500ml) water until smooth. Pour the mixture through a strainer lined with a fine cloth into a large bowl. Keep any blended nuts left behind for another use (see tips).

Vanilla nut milk

PREP TIME **10 MINUTES + STANDING** | MAKES **2 CUPS (500ML)**

Make nut milk on left using $1/2$ cup almonds and $1/2$ cup cashews. Split a vanilla bean lengthways, scrape the seeds into the milk; stir to combine.

Spiced nut milk

PREP TIME **15 MINUTES + STANDING** | MAKES **2 CUPS (500ML)**

Make the basic nut milk on left using 1 cup pecans. Stir in cinnamon sticks, star anise, and saffron threads. Stand; strain before using.

TIPS

- Using skinless or blanched nuts will create a whiter coloured milk.
- Using a high-powered blender will create a smoother textured milk.
- Dry out the strained, blended nuts on an oven tray in a 150°C/300°F oven. Sprinkle on your breakfast cereal or add to curries and pastes.

CLOCKWISE from top

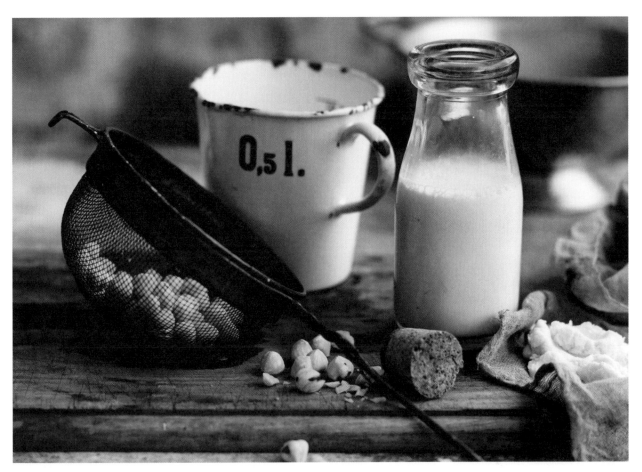

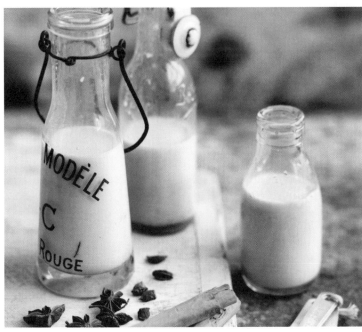

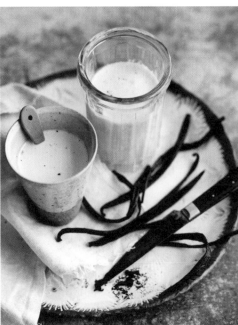

Baked ricotta pudding with orange and date salad

LACTO-OVO VEGETARIAN | PREP + COOK TIME **1 HOUR + COOLING & REFRIGERATION** | SERVES **4**

The pairing of orange and dates is classic Middle Eastern flavouring, which perfectly complements these creamy baked ricotta cheesecakes. This stunning desert will enhance any dinner party menu.

1 medium orange (240g)

1 medium blood orange (240g)

600g ricotta

3 eggs

1/3 cup (80ml) pure maple syrup

1/2 tsp ground cinnamon

4 fresh dates (80g), seeded, torn

2 tbsp pine nuts, toasted

fresh thyme sprigs, to serve

orange syrup

1/2 cup (125ml) freshly squeezed orange juice

2 tablespoons pure maple syrup

1 cinnamon stick

1/2 tsp fresh thyme leaves

1 Preheat oven 180°C (160°C fan/350°F/Gas 4). Grease four 3/4 cup (180ml), 10cm ovenproof dishes.

2 Finely grate the rind from the orange; you need 2 teaspoons. Cut the top and bottom from the orange and blood orange; cut off the white pith, following the curve of the fruit. Holding the orange, cut down both sides of the white membrane to release each segment. Cut the blood orange into thick slices. Set aside.

3 Process the ricotta, eggs, syrup, cinnamon, and orange rind until smooth. Pour the mixture evenly into the dishes.

4 Bake the puddings for 20 minutes or until the centre is just firm to touch. Cool to room temperature. Refrigerate for at least 1 hour or until cold.

5 Meanwhile, to make the orange syrup, bring the ingredients to the boil in a small saucepan. Reduce heat to low; simmer for 10 minutes or until syrupy. Refrigerate for 1 hour or until cold. Remove the cinnamon stick.

6 Serve the puddings topped with the orange segments, dates, syrup, pine nuts, and thyme sprigs.

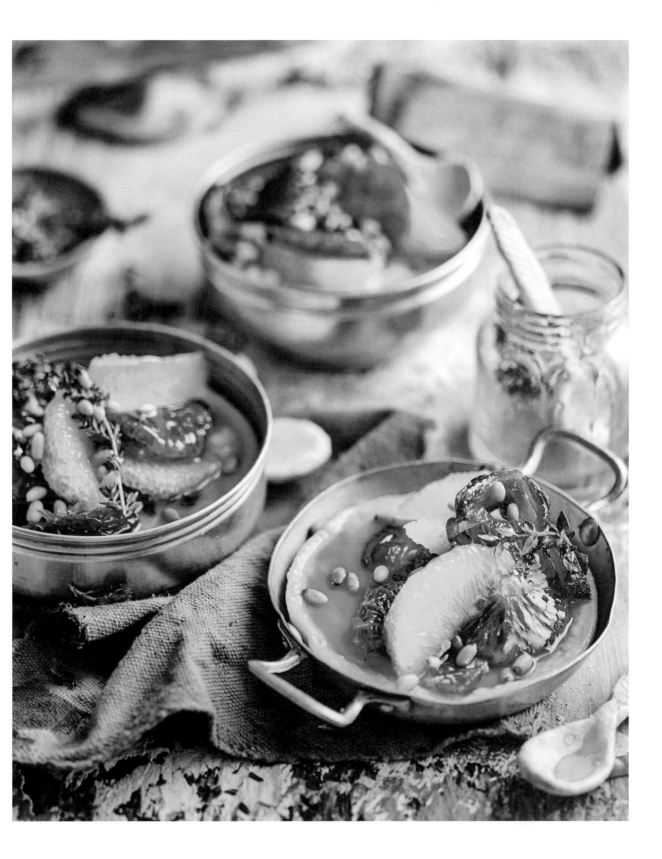

Gluten-free orange and white chocolate blondie

LACTO-OVO VEGETARIAN | PREP + COOK TIME **1 HOUR + COOLING** | MAKES **16 PIECES**

Blondies, sometimes referred to as blonde brownies, are rich, sweet dessert bars.
This buttery, nutty version is sprinkled with pistachios and finished to golden perfection.
Serve drizzled with honey.

150g white chocolate, coarsely chopped

100g butter, chopped

²/₃ cup (150g) caster sugar

2 eggs, lightly beaten

2 tsp finely grated orange rind

³/₄ cup (100g) gluten-free plain flour

¹/₂ cup (75g) tapioca flour

¹/₃ cup (50g) brown rice flour

¹/₂ cup (60g) almond meal (ground almonds)

¹/₃ cup (45g) coarsely chopped pistachios

¹/₄ cup (90g) honey

1   Preheat oven to 180°C (160°C fan/350°F/Gas 4). Grease a deep 19cm square cake pan; line the bottom and sides with baking paper.

2   Stir the chocolate and butter in a medium saucepan over a low heat for 5 minutes or until the chocolate melts and the mixture is smooth. Remove from the heat. Cool for 5 minutes.

3   Stir the sugar into the chocolate mixture; the mixture may appear split at this stage, however it will come together once the dry ingredients are added. Add the egg and orange rind; stir to combine. Stir in the sifted flours and almond meal until combined. Pour into the pan; sprinkle with pistachios.

4   Bake the blondie for 40 minutes or until a skewer inserted in the centre comes out clean. Drizzle the hot blondie with honey; cool in the pan before cutting into 16 squares.

TIP

Blondie can be made up to 3 days ahead; store in an airtight container.

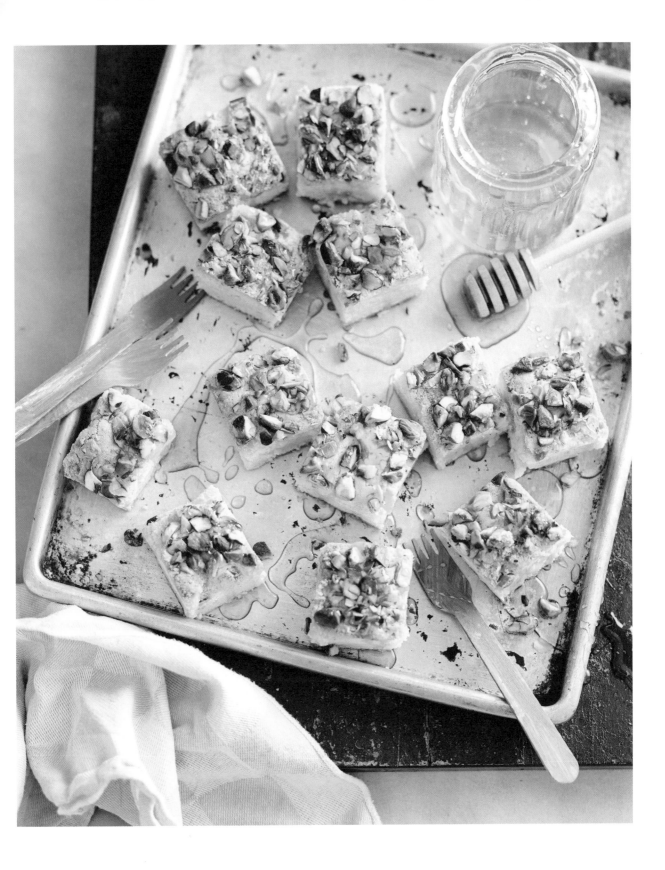

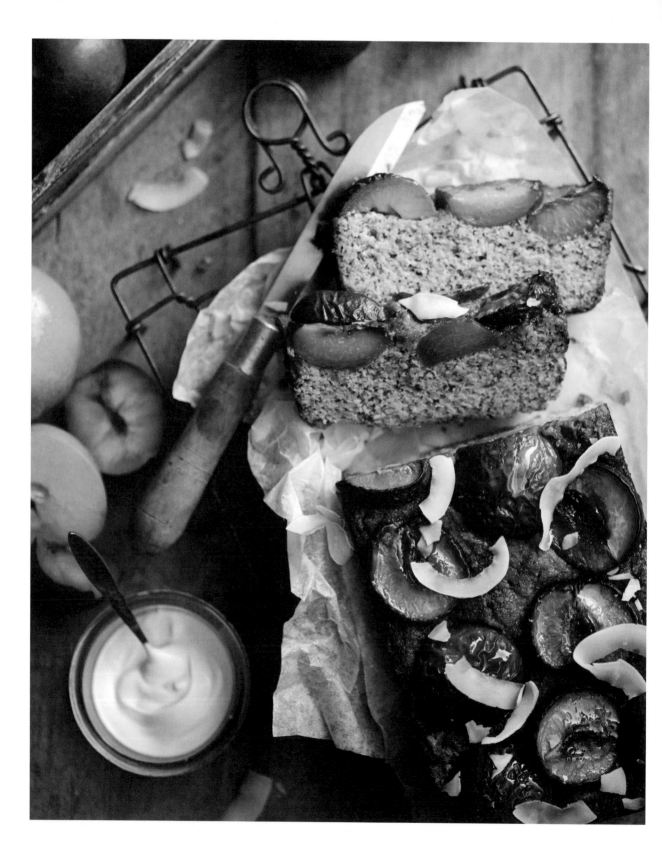

Flourless almond, plum, and orange blossom loaf

OVO VEGETARIAN | PREP + COOK TIME **1 HOURS 45 MINUTES** | SERVES **6**

Using no flour makes this a lighter, gluten-free alternative to traditional loaves. You can also make this loaf with other stone fruit such as small peaches or apricots. Best served with a warm pot of tea.

2 medium green apples (300g), coarsely grated

2 eggs, lightly beaten

¼ cup (60ml) unsweetened almond milk

2 tbsp raw honey or pure maple syrup

2 tsp vanilla extract

1 tsp orange blossom water

2 cups (240g) almond meal (ground almonds)

2 tsp gluten-free baking powder

5 small plums (375g), halved

2 tsp raw honey or pure maple syrup, extra

2 tbsp flaked coconut, toasted

1 Preheat oven to 160°C (140°C fan/325°F/Gas 3). Lightly grease a 10.5cm x 21cm x 6cm (base measurement) loaf pan; line the bottom and long sides with baking paper.

2 Combine the apple, egg, almond milk, honey, vanilla, and orange blossom water in a large bowl. Add the almond meal and baking powder; stir until just combined.

3 Spread the mixture into the pan, level the surface; top with plums, cut-side up, pressing them slightly into the batter. Drizzle with extra honey.

4 Bake for 1½ hours or until a skewer inserted into the centre comes out clean. Top with the coconut and serve warm.

TIP

You may need to cover the loaf loosely with baking paper during the last 10 minutes of baking to prevent overbrowning.

Banana and coffee cake with caramel sauce

LACTO-OVO VEGETARIAN | PREP + COOK TIME **1 HOUR 45 MINUTES** | SERVES **12**

This decadent cake takes the sweetness of bananas and the hit of coffee to produce the perfect teatime treat or after-dinner delight. Best served warm out of the oven and drizzled with indulgent caramel sauce.

185g butter, softened, chopped

1 cup (245g) granulated stevia

3 eggs

2¼ cups (335g) self-raising flour

¼ tsp salt

¾ tsp bicarbonate of soda

1½ tsp ground cinnamon

2 cups (560g) mashed ripe banana (see tips)

2 tsp vanilla extract

¾ cup (200g) sour cream

1 cup (100g) walnuts, roasted, chopped

¼ cup (60ml) boiling water

3 tsp espresso coffee granules

caramel sauce

⅔ cup (200g) rice malt syrup

125g butter, softened, chopped

⅓ cup (80ml) thickened (double) cream

1 Preheat oven to 180°C (160°C fan/350°F/Gas 4). Grease and line a deep 22cm (9in) round cake pan with baking paper.

2 Beat the butter and stevia in a small bowl with an electric mixer until pale and fluffy. Beat in the eggs, one at a time, until just combined. Transfer the mixture to a large bowl. Stir the sifted dry ingredients, banana, vanilla, sour cream, walnuts, and combined water and coffee into the butter mixture. Spread the mixture into the pan.

3 Bake the cake for 1¼ hours or until a skewer inserted into the centre comes out clean. Leave the cake in the pan for 5 minutes before turning, top-side up, onto a wire rack to cool.

4 Meanwhile, make the caramel sauce. Place the syrup in a small saucepan over a medium heat, bring to the boil; boil for 12 minutes or until slightly darker golden in colour, and the surface is covered with bubbles. Immediately add butter and cream; stir until the mixture is smooth.

5 Serve cake with the caramel sauce.

TIPS

- You will need about 4 large bananas to make 2 cups of mashed banana.
- The cake can be made a day ahead; store in an airtight container at room temperature in a cool place.

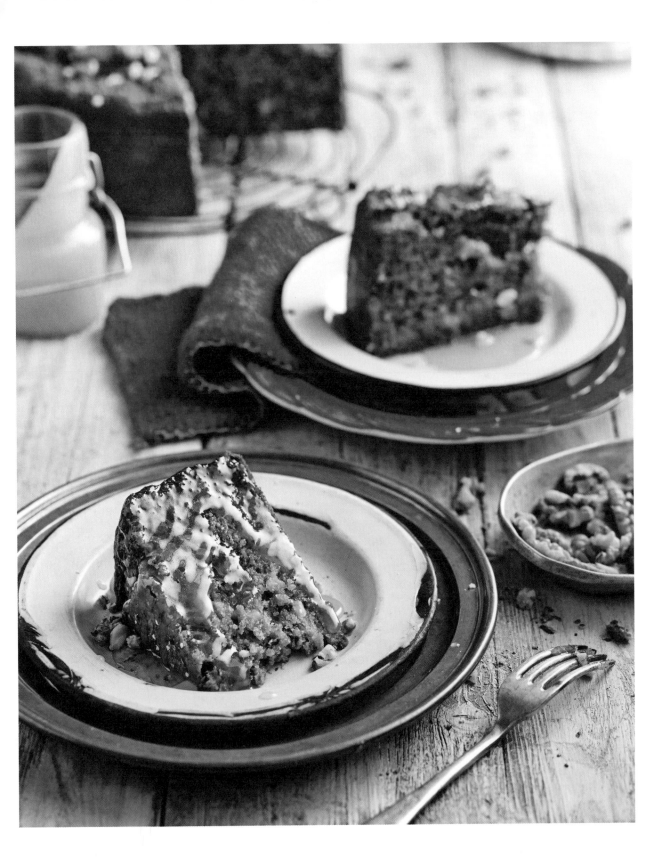

Conversion chart

A note on Australian measures

- One Australian metric measuring cup holds approximately 250ml.

- One Australian metric tablespoon holds 20ml.

- One Australian metric teaspoon holds 5ml.

- The difference between one country's measuring cups and another's is within a two- or three-teaspoon variance, and should not affect your cooking results.

- North America, New Zealand, and the United Kingdom use a 15ml tablespoon.

Using measures in this book

- All cup and spoon measurements are level.

- The most accurate way of measuring dry ingredients is to weigh them.

- When measuring liquids, use a clear glass or plastic jug with metric markings.

- We use large eggs with an average weight of 60g.

Dry measures

metric	imperial
15g	$1/2$oz
30g	1oz
60g	2oz
90g	3oz
125g	4oz ($1/4$lb)
155g	5oz
185g	6oz
220g	7oz
250g	8oz ($1/2$lb)
280g	9oz
315g	10oz
345g	11oz
375g	12oz ($3/4$lb)
410g	13oz
440g	14oz
470g	15oz
500g	16oz (1lb)
750g	24oz ($1^1/2$lb)
1kg	32oz (2lb)

Liquid measures

metric	imperial
30ml	1 fluid oz
60ml	2 fluid oz
100ml	3 fluid oz
125ml	4 fluid oz
150ml	5 fluid oz
190ml	6 fluid oz
250ml	8 fluid oz
300ml	10 fluid oz
500ml	16 fluid oz
600ml	20 fluid oz
1000ml (1 litre)	$1^3/4$ pints

Length measures

metric	imperial
3mm	$1/8$in
6mm	$1/4$in
1cm	$1/2$in
2cm	$3/4$in
2.5cm	1in
5cm	2in
6cm	$2^1/2$in
8cm	3in
10cm	4in
13cm	5in
15cm	6in
18cm	7in
20cm	8in
22cm	9in
25cm	10in
28cm	11in
30cm	12in (1ft)

Oven temperatures

The oven temperatures in this book are for conventional ovens; if you have a fan-forced oven, decrease the temperature by 10–20 degrees.

	°C (Celsius)	°F (Fahrenheit)
Very slow	120	250
Slow	150	300
Moderately slow	160	325
Moderate	180	350
Moderately hot	200	400
Hot	220	425
Very hot	240	475

Index

Acknowledgments

DK would like to thank Sophia Young, Simone Aquilina, Amanda Chebatte, and Georgia Moore for their assistance in making this book.

The Australian Women's Weekly Test Kitchen in Sydney, Australia has developed, tested and photographed the recipes in this book.